Tumor Microenvironment - New Insights

Edited by Ahmed Lasfar

Published in London, United Kingdom

Tumor Microenvironment - New Insights
http://dx.doi.org/10.5772/intechopen.102243
Edited by Ahmed Lasfar

Contributors
Elisa Frullanti, Maria Palmieri, Jer-Yen Yang, Xing-Guo Li, Sajna Panolan, Srinivas Govindarajulu, S. Kalpana, Valarmathi Srinivasan, Joseph Maria Adaikalam, Yi Lu, Adith Kotha, Chikezie O. Madu, Catherine T. Flores, Dan Jin, Laura Falceto Font, Anyu Gu, Gaetana Messina, Mary Bove, Giorgia Opromolla, Vincenzo Di Filippo, Mario Pirozzi, Marianna Caterino, Sergio Facchini, Alessia Zotta, Giovanni Vicidomini, Mario Santini, Alfonso Fiorelli, Fortunato Ciardiello, Morena Fasano

First published in London, United Kingdom, 2023 by IntechOpen
IntechOpen is the global imprint of INTECHOPEN LIMITED, registered in England and Wales, registration number: 11086078, 5 Princes Gate Court, London, SW7 2QJ, United Kingdom

British Library Cataloguing-in-Publication Data
A catalogue record for this book is available from the British Library

Additional hard and PDF copies can be obtained from orders@intechopen.com

Tumor Microenvironment - New Insights
Edited by Ahmed Lasfar
p. cm.
Print ISBN 978-1-83969-379-3
Online ISBN 978-1-83969-380-9
eBook (PDF) ISBN 978-1-83969-381-6

For EU product safety concerns:
IN TECH d.o.o., Prolaz Marije Krucifikse Kozulić 3, 51000 Rijeka, Croatia,
info@intechopen.com or visit our website at intechopen.com.

Meet the editor

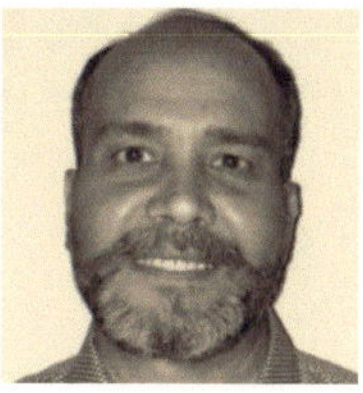

Dr. Ahmed Lasfar is a faculty member at Rutgers University and a full member of the Rutgers Cancer Institute of New Jersey, USA. He is an editor and board member of several international journals and books. Dr. Lasfar is a scientific adviser and consultant to the pharmaceutical industry and a member of several medical and scientific societies. He graduated in Medical and Applied Science (BS/MD) and obtained a Ph.D. in Immunology from Paris Diderot University, France. Dr. Lasfar completed his postdoctoral training in cancer immunology at Robert Wood Johnson Medical School, New Jersey, USA.

Contents

Preface

The tumor microenvironment (TME) is a crucial aspect of all cancer types. It is well established now that TME plays an important role in both the control and the development of solid tumors. The histology of TME consists of a variety of normal resident and recruited cells, which are involved in concise and dynamic interactions with cancer cells. These interactions, which occur via released factors or cell-to-cell contact, are fundamental in tumor-induced suppression and metastatic dissemination of cancer cells, ultimately leading to morbidity and/or mortality for most cancer patients. Considerable progress has been made in understanding the mechanisms by which the TME contributes to the inhibition or promotion of cancer, enabling the emergence of a range of novel targeted therapies. In addition to stroma-targeted strategies, checkpoint inhibitor-based immunotherapy has emerged as a new treatment of choice for many advanced cancers. However, many cancer patients remain resistant to current therapies, necessitating the development of more innovative therapeutic strategies based on the identification of new targets and combining drugs that could counteract resistance. In this book, *Tumor Microenvironment – New Insights*, the authors highlight this aspect with chapters that describe and discuss innovative and impactful studies.

Prominent efforts and collaborations with leading experts in cancer were crucial in achieving this highly valuable book. We thank all the authors for their tremendous expertise and their exceptional quality in pointing out the crucial role of TME in cancer. Understanding and targeting TME constitutes a new hope for cancer patients, particularly those with advanced diseases.

Ahmed Lasfar
Department of Toxicology and Pharmacology,
Rutgers University,
NJ, USA

Section 1

Novel Diagnosis and Treatment of Cancer

Chapter 1

Liquid Biopsy: A New Strategy for Future Directions in Lung Cancer Treatment

Maria Palmieri and Elisa Frullanti

Abstract

The gold standard for cancer diagnosis has always been based on radiological imaging followed by surgical tissue biopsies for molecular testing and pathological examination and surgical resection to remove the tumoral mass when possible. However, the resulting information is a limited snapshot in space and time, which poorly reflects clonal heterogeneity or tumor evolution and metastasis. Over a decade since its inception, the ability to use non-invasive methods such as a liquid biopsy to analyze tumor biomarkers has transformed the vision of future cancer care into a better patient experience thanks to real-time monitoring and early diagnosis. The liquid biopsy essay is an effective tool for detecting cancers at an early stage, when there are very few tumor-derived materials circulating in the bloodstream, being a very sensitive technique. For this reason, liquid biopsy is particularly suitable for early-stage diagnosis (stage I or II) of lung cancer whose diagnosis often occurs in the final stages of the disease as well as monitoring cancer progression and driving target therapies.

Keywords: liquid biopsy, lung cancer, CfDNA, new strategies, Circulating Tumor DNA (CtDNA)

1. Introduction

1.1 An early opportunity to catch cancer

A cancer patient's torturous journey begins with formulating the diagnosis. The detection of tumor mass, the stage, and the molecular profile are all clues that lead to the proper treatment. The advent of new technologies allows us to deepen our knowledge of molecular data useful to physicians to guide them toward specific therapies.

Cancer is the World's second biggest killer after heart disease, in which some of the body's cells grow uncontrollably and spread to other parts of the body. Currently, 90% of cancer patients do not die from the primary tumor but are killed by its distant metastases. Current treatment of patients with metastatic cancer is generally driven by the molecular characteristics of the primary tumor. Detection and monitoring of the disease are carried out with tissue sampling in a common and invasive difficult way for patients with solid tumors. Recently, sequential peripheral blood tests have been introduced as a non-invasive technique, resulting in the use of liquid biopsy [1]. Liquid biopsy refers to a test, usually carried out from blood samples, to analyze tumor molecular biomarkers that can diagnose cancer and inform clinical decision-making [1].

Here, we will explore the possible molecular biomarkers that can be used:

- *The circulating tumor cells* (CTCs) are released from both primary and metastatic tumor sites into the bloodstream. Tumor cells are recognized by the shape and/or physical elements such as size, density, electric charges and deformability and biological characteristics, cell surface protein expression and viability [1]. CTCs have a short half-life, between 1 and 2.5 hours and the process by which the CTCs are released into the bloodstream is not yet well understood. Although their role in metastasis remains poorly undigested, it is highly probable that CTCs are the precursors of the different metastatic populations [2] even if there are less than 10 CTCs per 7.5 ml of blood [3]. For this reason, CTCs require detection and enrichment processes being caught through positive (which relies on antibodies capturing the surface tumor antigen expressed on the CTCs) or negative (removing the other blood components using size filtration) selection. CTCs can be analyzed in a multidimensional characterization, at protein, DNA, and RNA level.

- *The Circulating Tumor DNA* (CtDNA) is the fragmented tumoral DNA that can be detected in the bloodstream, derived from apoptotic and necrotic tumor cells. During the normal apoptosis processes (programmed cell death) or necrosis (cell trauma—premature death), the cell undergoes a series of morphological changes, and the chromatin is condensed and degraded into small fragments, approximately 200 bp in length, and released circulating in the blood. These DNA fragments are also known as cell-free DNA (cf-DNA) and can be acquired by isolating DNA from plasma or serum. Nowadays, next generation sequencing (NGS)-based analyses and digital PCR (dPCR)-based methods are the most frequently used to detect ctDNA.

The analytes mentioned above are the most studied as they are detected more easily alone or in combination, but exosomes, RNA, extracellular vesicles and, last but not least, methylation must also be counted among others.

To date, the gold standard for cancer analysis in clinical practice is tissue biopsy. This implies that, despite the advantages of liquid biopsy that immediately appear very clear, it is necessary to demonstrate that this non-invasive approach is actually better than the current one. The greatest limitation of all tissue biopsies is the lack of representativeness of tumor heterogeneity and plasticity. Tumors are highly heterogeneous, even down to the single cell level, and their characteristics change over time and under treatment pressure. The recovery of the sample through tissue biopsy is a highly invasive practice for the patient and is not easily repeatable over time, thus making the information of the data obsolete over time. For its part, the liquid biopsy can be defined as minimally invasive and allows the monitoring of the evolution of the tumor characteristics over time thanks to the possibility of being able to repeat the practice of blood sampling and in a sequential way also during the course of treatment (**Figure 1**).

Even if the initial approach leads us to think of using the liquid biopsy rather than the tissue biopsy, we should start thinking of starting to collect different data deriving from both approaches to really have clear and comprehensive information that guides cancer treatment.

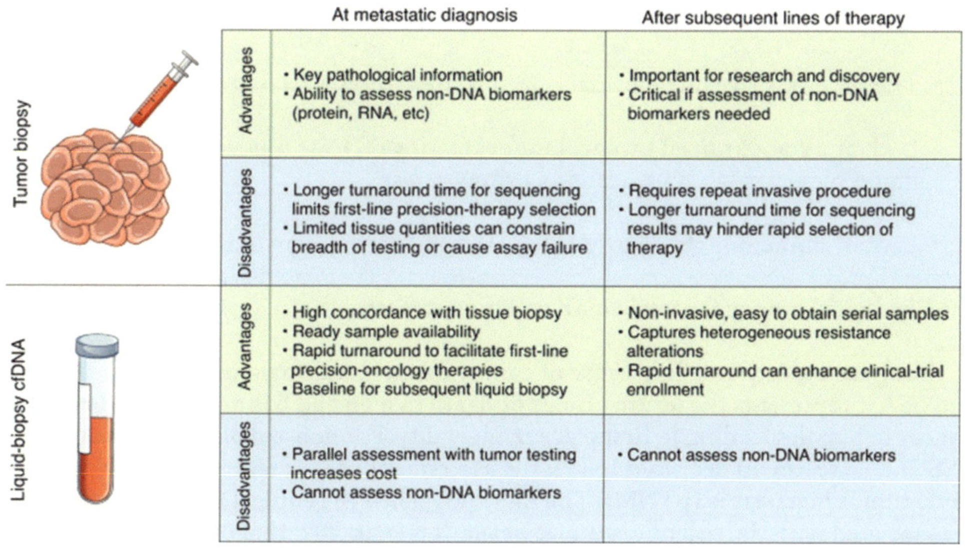

Figure 1.
Liquid biopsy versus tumor biopsy for clinical-trial recruitment [4].

1.2 The potential use of liquid biopsy through the patient's journey

Thanks to the sensitivity and specificity achievable with high-depth sequencing, liquid biopsy can be used for the early diagnosis of cancer, and in the next future also as a screening in healthy people. To justify this use, however, it is necessary to demonstrate that the tests are better than those currently in use. Indeed, some studies have shown that ctDNA analysis was able to diagnose lung cancer in the early stages (stage I or II) [5], as well as the detection of some mutations (i.e. *TP53* or *KRAS* genes) which is possible many years earlier, when the individual is still asymptomatic, compared to the time of the classic diagnosis [6].

Additionally, liquid biopsy can be extremely useful in detecting residual molecular disease (MRD) after treatment. In fact, it is very common that after specific medical treatments the current radiological imaging techniques are not able to detect the MRD [7] responsible for relapse.

However, before liquid biopsy enters the clinical routine, several clinical trials are needed for normalization and experimentation and would help answer several unsuspended questions. In fact, clinical trials allow facing challenges such as [8]:

- reproducibility and sensitivity.
- distinguish positive results from negative results.
- biomarker efficacy.

A recent study [9] shows that at the moment the analyses of cfDNA are mainly included in clinical trials for cancers that have a higher incidence and mortality such as lung, breast, and colon cancer. Additionally, the study found some main drawbacks that were common among several trials that risk demoralizing and/or confusing the patient:

- The lack of consensus on terminology
- The false-positive rate: normal cells may have tumor-related mutations
- Lack of a standardized protocol for evaluating cfDNA: hinders the routine use of liquid biopsy in laboratories as an ordinary test
- Lack of numerous cohorts that allow the standardization of the data

1.3 The liquid biopsy for non-small cell lung cancer

Lung cancer is the leading cause of cancer death in industrialized countries. In the USA it represents the leading cause of death in men and has now passed breast cancer in females leading to first place in mortality. For non-small cell lung cancer (NSCLC), treatment decisions follow the assessment of the staging of pathological node tumor metastases (pTNM). The more advanced the clinical stage, the more this is associated with the risk of death. However, it is estimated that only 40% of patients have stage 2–3 and have a minimal residual disease (MRD), and this means that the remaining 60% are likely to be over-treated with the possibility of giving rise to high toxicity risks. Somatic molecular alterations in NSCLC can lead to oncogene activation through multiple genetic mechanisms (point mutations, insertions, deletions, gene rearrangements, etc.) and the treatment of cancer has thus evolved from broad chemotherapeutic approaches to therapies targeted against specific molecular abnormalities that drive tumor growth. A robust and accurate assessment of molecular alterations within tumor cells is mandatory in routine clinical practice to determine which patients are suitable for these targeted therapies.

The TRACERx study (Tracking Cancer Evolution through Therapy) is a British national observational study for patients with NSCLC who have undergone surgery. Through this study, they try to evaluate the natural history of the evolution of the disease in order to understand the biology of MRD when it is impossible to access a tissue biopsy again. By monitoring 30 tumor variants, they were able to identify cases of disease recurrence by detecting MRD prior to clinical surveillance. They are currently looking to implement over 200 variants and limit of detection (LOD) of the technique in well over 1000 plasma samples. Therefore, thanks to this pioneering study it is possible to use two approaches:

- the first allows using the ctDNA as a biomarker after the surgery of a patient affected by NSCLC in two temporal points in order to detect the MRD and to enroll the patient in combined therapy;
- the second approach is MRD surveillance to identify those patients who already have a relapse in order to intervene immediately with the therapy in a time.

Historically, the first clinical application of liquid biopsy in advanced NSCLC was the detection of *EGFR* mutations (**Figure 2**). From these pioneering studies, the scientists moved on to the analysis of next-generation sequencing (NGS) which allowed expanding the investigation to other driver mutations as well, that could provide prognostic and predictive information [10].

The first methods used were those of RT-PCR (real-time PCR) capable of detecting *EGFR* mutations and at the moment the only one approved by the FDA for the

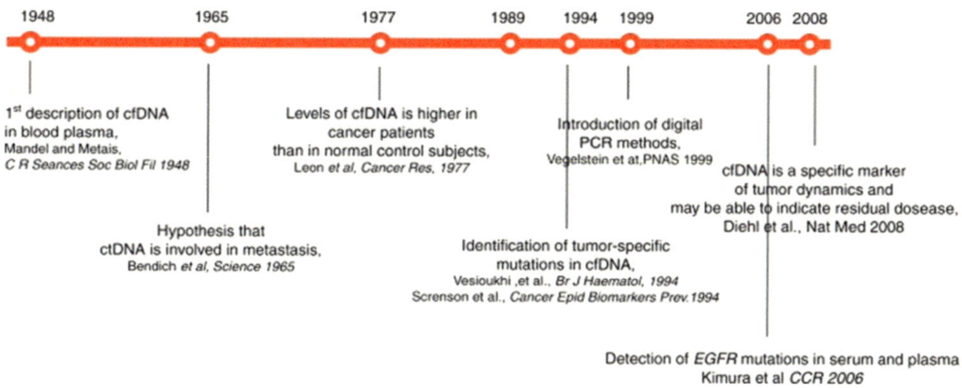

Figure 2.
Timeline of the development of liquid biopsy [10].

detection of the T790M resistance mutation of the *EGFR* gene [11]. Indeed, in 2016, the Food and Drug Administration (FDA) approved the liquid biopsy test for patients with NSCLC to verify EGFR-targeted therapy, while a European consortium from the European Liquid Biopsy Academy (ELBA) using biomarkers such as ctDNA, CTC, exosomes, and tumor educated platelets (TEP) [12].

Currently, ESMO guidelines recommend testing at least *EGFR* mutations, *BRAF* mutations, *ALK* fusions, *ROS-1* fusions, *MET* exon 14 skipping mutations, *RET* rearrangements and PD-L1 expression levels in non-squamous advanced NSCLC [13]. This panel could be further implemented considering *KRAS* mutations, *HER2* mutations, *MET* amplification, and *NTRK* rearrangements [13].

2. Conclusion

In conclusion, we can state that the liquid biopsy is significantly helping the management of patients with lung cancer by crossing the threshold of the use of off-label drugs in therapeutic pathways [14], but we must be aware that liquid biopsy cannot replace the PDL-1 expression assay for investigation of the tumor immune microenvironment, as well as cytological analysis of tissue biopsy. Therefore, in order to obtain the most complete treatment possible, we must consider liquid biopsy not as a competitive approach to the already existing ones, but as another valid mutation detection option.

Declaration

The authors have no conflicts of interest.

Author details

Maria Palmieri[1,2] and Elisa Frullanti[1,2*]

1 Department of Medical Biotechnologies, University of Siena, Siena, Italy

2 Med Biotech Hub and Competence Center, Department of Medical Biotechnologies, University of Siena, Siena, Italy

*Address all correspondence to: elisa.frullanti@dbm.unisi.it

References

[1] Pantel K, Alix-Panabières C. Circulating tumour cells in cancer patients: Challenges and perspectives. Trends in Molecular Medicine. 2010;**16**(9):398-406. DOI: 10.1016/j.molmed.2010.07.001

[2] Meng S, Tripathy D, Frenkel E. et al, Circulating tumor cells in patients with breast cancer dormancy. Clinical Cancer Research. 2004;**10**(24):8152-8162. DOI: 10.1158/1078-0432.ccr-04-1110

[3] Crowley E, Di Nicolantonio F, Loupakis F, Bardelli A. Liquid biopsy: Monitoring cancer-genetics in the blood. Nature Reviews. Clinical Oncology. 2013;**10**(8):472-484. DOI: 10.1038/nrclinonc.2013.110 Epub 2013 Jul 9

[4] Corcoran RB. Liquid biopsy versus tumor biopsy for clinical-trial recruitment. Nature Medicine. 2020;**26**:1815-1816. DOI: 10.1038/s41591-020-01169-6

[5] Phallen J, Sausen M, Adleff V, et al. Direct detection of early-stage cancers using circulating tumor DNA. Science Translational Medicine. 2017;**9**(403):aan2415. DOI: 10.1126/scitranslmed

[6] Gormally E, Vineis P, Matullo G, et al. TP53 and KRAS2 mutations in plasma DNA of healthy subjects and subsequent cancer occurrence: A prospective study. Cancer Research. 2006;**66**(13):6871-6876. DOI: 10.1158/0008-5472.can-05-4556

[7] Pantel K, Alix-Panabières C. Liquid biopsy and minimal residual disease—Latest advances and implications for cure. Nature Reviews Clinical Oncology. 2019;**16**(7):409-424. DOI: 10.1038/s41571-019-0187-3

[8] Lustberg M, Stover D, Chalmers J. Implementing liquid biopsies in clinical trials. The Cancer Journal. 2018;**24**(2):61-64. DOI: 10.1097/ppo.0000000000000309

[9] Cisneros-Villanueva M, Hidalgo-Pérez L, Rios-Romero M, et al. Cell-free DNA analysis in current cancer clinical trials: A review. British Journal of Cancer. 2022;**126**(3):391-400. DOI: 10.1038/s41416-021-01696-0

[10] Bonanno L, Dal Maso A, Pavan A, et al. Liquid biopsy and non-small cell lung cancer: Are we looking at the tip of the iceberg? British Journal of Cancer. 2022. DOI: 10.1038/s41416-022-01777-8

[11] Sacher AG, Paweletz C, Dahlberg SE, Alden RS, O'Connell A, Feeney N, et al. Prospective validation of rapid plasma genotyping for the detection of EGFR and KRAS mutations in advanced lung cancer. JAMA Oncology. 2016;**2**:1014

[12] Revelo AE, Martin A, Velasquez R, Kulandaisamy PC, Bustamante J, Keshishyan S, et al. Liquid biopsy for lung cancers: An update on recent developments. Annals of Translational Medicine. 2019;**7**(15):349. DOI: 10.21037/atm.2019.03.28

[13] Planchard D, Popat S, Kerr K, Novello S, Smit EF, Faivre-Finn C, et al. Metastatic non-small cell lung cancer: ESMO clinical practice guidelines for diagnosis, treatment and follow-up. Annals of Oncology. 2018;**29**:iv192-iv237

[14] Danesi R, Fogli S, Indraccolo S, Del Re M, Dei Tos AP, Leoncini L, et al. Druggable targets meet oncogenic drivers: Opportunities and limitations of target-based classification of tumors and the role of molecular tumor boards. ESMO Open. Apr 2021;**6**(2):100040

Chapter 2

Minimally Invasive Surgery for the Management of Lung Cancer

Gaetana Messina, Mary Bove, Giorgia Opromolla, Vincenzo Di Filippo, Mario Pirozzi, Marianna Caterino, Sergio Facchini, Alessia Zotta, Giovanni Vicidomini, Mario Santini, Alfonso Fiorelli, Fortunato Ciardiello and Morena Fasano

Abstract

Lung cancer is the leading cause of cancer-related death and the most diagnosed cancer. The treatment of Non-Small Cell Lung Cancer (NSCLC) depends on clinical staging. Surgical radical resection is recommended for patients with stage 1 or 2 of disease and represents the treatment of choice. In the last decades, the surgical approach for lung cancer changed moving from an open approach to a minimally invasive approach, represented by Video Assisted Thoracic Surgery (VATS) and Robot-Assisted Thoracic Surgery (RATS). In this chapter, we illustrate the characteristics of lung cancer, the diagnosis, the classification, the staging and the preoperative evaluation. Then we focus on the surgical treatment of lung cancer and on how it has changed during the years. We explain the open approach represented by the traditional posterolateral thoracotomy and by the muscle-sparing thoracotomy. We illustrate VATS approach and evolution: from the hybrid approach to the pure VATS that can be triportal, biportal or even uniportal. Then, we focus on RATS approach, characterized by the use of multiple ports in the same intercostal space and how it evolved toward the uniportal approach. The objective is to combine the advantage of uniportal VATS (lower postoperative pain, enhanced recovery) and RATS (better visualization, more degrees of movements).

Keywords: NSCLC, thoracic surgery, VATS, RATS, Uniportal, minimally invasive surgery

1. Introduction

1.1 Epidemiology

Lung cancer is one of the main causes of death in several countries. The incidence of lung cancer is 3% in men and 1% in women. 236.740 new cases of lung cancer and 130.180 deaths have been recorded in 2022 [1]. 5-years survival rate is 21.7%, in particular it is 15% for men and 19% for women [2]. It represents the first cause of death for tumor for men and the second for women.

Cigarette smoking is the main risk factor for lung cancer, because of its carcinogenic chemicals. Relative risk of lung cancer is related to number of cigarettes smoked per day, years of smoking and level of tar in cigarettes. Exposed non-smokers also have an increased relative risk of developing lung cancer.

Many agents, such as asbestos, beryllium, cadmium, chromium, diesel fumes nickel, are known as carcinogens. They increase the risk of lung cancer in exposed people, especially in smokers. About 80–90% of lung cancer is caused by smoking. The risk of lung cancer is increased in ex-smokers than in never smokers [3]. Some genetic factors, such as overexpression of Epidermal Growth Factor (EGFR), are related to the development of non-small cell lung cancer (NSCLC) [4].

1.2 Lung cancer screening

The National Lung Screening Trial (NLST) was the first trial to demonstrate that early diagnosis of lung cancer with annual low-dose CT scan in individuals with high-risk factors reduces the mortality rate related to this disease of 20% compared to chest radiographs. In this trial, individuals with high-risk factors were current or former smokers with a 30 or more pack-year smoking history, 55 to 74 years of age with no evidence of lung cancer [5]. Different organizations such as European Respiratory Society (ERS), European Society of Radiology (ESR), European Society of Thoracic Surgeons (ESTS), European Alliance for Personalized Medicine (EAPM), European Society of Medical Oncology (ESMO) e Swiss University Hospitals recommend lung cancer screening with low-dose CT scan. Anyway, low-dose CT screening and follow-up do not substitute smoking cessation.

1.3 Classification and prognostic factors

World Health Organization (WHO) divides lung cancer into two main categories non-small cell lung cancer (NSCLC) and small cell lung cancer (SCLC). The 80% of lung cancer is represented by NSCLC. It is divided into two groups: (1) non-squamous: adenocarcinoma, large-cell carcinoma and other subtypes; (2) squamous cell carcinoma [6]. **Table 1** summarizes WHO classification of lung cancer.

In the last decades, the histological definitions of NSCLS become critical for the development of new therapies based on the histotype. Diagnosis can be obtained with morphological criteria based on hematoxylin and eosin stain or specific stains, such as May-Grunwald-Giemsa, but immunohistochemistry is crucial for the definition of poorly differentiated NSCLC or Not Otherwise Specified (NOS).

Immunohistochemical investigation can be conducted both on histological or cytological samples.

The study of the molecular characteristics of lung cancer, the individuation of disease-associated mutations (EGFR mutations) or immune biomarkers (PD-L1) is crucial for target therapy, that is effective in patients with specific mutations [7].

1.4 Clinical manifestations

Lung cancer can manifest with symptoms like cough, dyspnea, pain, fatigue or hemoptysis. Symptoms related to advanced stages of disease are weight loss, pleural effusion, dysphagia, lymphadenopathy, paraneoplastic syndromes [8].

Epithelial tumors
Papillomas
Squamous cell papilloma, NOS Squamous cell papilloma, inverted Glandular papilloma Mixed squamous cell and glandular papilloma
Adenomas
Sclerosing pneumocytoma Alveolar adenoma Papillary adenoma Bronchiolar adenoma/ciliated muconodular papillary tumor Mucinous cystadenoma Mucous gland adenoma
Precursor glandular lesion
Atypical adenomatous hyperplasia Adenocarcinoma in situ Adenocarcinoma in situ, nonmucinous Adenocarcinoma in situ, mucinous
Adenocarcinomas
Minimally invasive adenocarcinoma Minimally invasive adenocarcinoma, nonmucinous Minimally invasive adenocarcinoma, mucinous Invasive non-mucinous adenocarcinoma Lepidic adenocarcinoma Acinar adenocarcinoma Papillary adenocarcinoma Micropapillary adenocarcinoma Solid adenocarcinoma Invasive mucinous adenocarcinoma Mixed invasive mucinous and nonmucinous adenocarcinoma
Colloid adenocarcinoma
Fetal adenocarcinoma
Adenocarcinoma, enteric type
Adenocarcinoma, NOS
Squamous precursor lesion Squamous cell carcinoma, NOS Squamous cell carcinoma, keratinizing Squamous cell carcinoma, nonkeratizing Basaloid squamous cell carcinoma Lymphoepithelial carcinoma
Large cell carcinoma
Adenosquamous carcinoma
Sarcomatoid carcinomas Pleomorphic carcinoma Giant cell carcinoma Spindle cell carcinoma Pulmonary blastoma Carcinosarcoma
Other epithelial tumors NUT carcinoma Thoracic SMARCA4-deficient undifferentiated tumor
Salivary gland-type tumors Pleomorphic adenoma Adenoid cystic carcinoma Mucoepidermoid carcinoma Hyalinizing clear cell carcinoma Myoepithelioma Myoepithelial carcinoma
Lung neuroendocrine neoplasms
Precursor lesion Diffuse idiopathic neuroendocrine cell hyperplasia
Neuroendocrine tumors Carcinoid tumor, NOS/neuroendocrine tumor, NOS Typical carcinoid/neuroendocrine tumor, grade 1 Atypical carcinoid/neuroendocrine tumor, grade 2
Neuroendocrine carcinomas Small cell carcinoma Combined small cell carcinoma Large cell neuroendocrine carcinoma Combined large cell neuroendocrine carcinoma

Tumors of ectopic tissues
Melanoma
Meningioma
Mesenchymal tumors specific to the lung
Pulmonary hamartoma
Chondroma
Diffuse lymphangiomatosis
Pleuropulmonary blastoma
Intimal sarcoma
Congenital peribronchial myofibroblastic tumor
Pulmonary myxoid sarcoma with EWSR1-CREB1 fusion
PEComatous tumors Lymphangioleiomyomatosi PEComa, benign PEComa, malignant
Hematolymphoid tumors
MALT lymphoma
Diffuse large B-cell lymphoma, NOS
Lymphomatoid granulomatosis, NOS Lymphomatoid granulomatosis, grade 1 Lymphomatoid granulomatosis, grade 2 Lymphomatoid granulomatosis, grade 3
Intravascular large B-cell lymphoma
Langerhans cell histiocytosis
Erdheim-Chester disease

Table 1.
WHO classification of lung cancer.

2. Diagnosis

Clinical suspicion of lung cancer is based on clinical evaluation and history (smoking history, symptoms, age, previous cancer history, family history, other lung disease). Chest X-ray is generally the first investigation performed. Incidental radiological finding of a suspected lung cancer is frequent and it often presents as a solitary or peripheral nodule. Suspicion findings have to be investigated by CT with contrast (**Figure 1**). Radiological features of the pulmonary nodule that suggest the diagnosis of lung cancer are: size, shape and density. The size of the neoformation and especially its growth over time is closely related to the risk of malignancy. However, the doubling of the volume of the nodule in less than 7 days indicates benign lesion (inflammation/infection). Spiculation, irregular margins and pleural retraction are associated with an increased risk of malignancy. Density of the neoformation can be homogeneous or inhomogeneous and varies from solid lesions to "ground glass" or partially solid lesions [9, 10].

Positron Emission Tomography/Computed Tomography (PET/CT) is playing a significant role as a potential diagnosis and staging test in patients with non-small cell lung cancer (NSCLC) [11] and allows, moreover, to direct the biopsy on suspect areas with elevated glucidic metabolism, increasing the likelihood of reaching a diagnostic result.

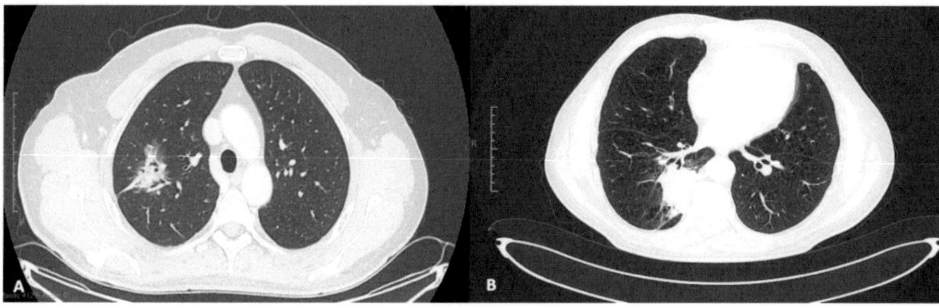

Figure 1.
Examples of lung cancer at CT scan: (A) tumor located at right upper lobe; (B) tumor located at right lower lobe.

Tissue diagnosis employs several techniques:

- Sputum cytology
- Bronchoalveolar Lavage (BAL)
- Image-guided transthoracic needle core biopsy or fine needle aspiration
- Bronchoscopy with biopsy or Transbronchial Needle Sspiration (TBNA)
- EBUS-guided biopsy
- EUS-guided biopsy

If a preoperative tissue diagnosis cannot be obtained, the alternative is intraoperative diagnosis (wedge resection or needle biopsy). The choice of diagnostic technique mainly depends on the location of the lesion (central or peripheral) but also on the size of the tumor and the clinical condition of the patient [12, 13].

In case of abnormal mediastinal and/or hilar lymph nodes at CT and/or PET, needle aspiration EBUS or EUS-guided is recommended. If malignant nodal involvement is not found by this techniques, surgical staging is recommended [12].

3. Staging and TNM classification

Lung cancer staging is necessary to establish the prognosis and the therapeutic program. Staging involves performing a contrast-enhanced CT scan of the chest and upper abdomen to determine local invasiveness, nodal involvement and distant metastasis, particularly in the liver and adrenal glands. The evaluation of these parameters defines the staging of the neoplastic disease according to the TNM system. TNM classification is universally accepted and routinely applied in clinical practice. The T category describes the size and the extension of the primary tumor; the N category defines regional lymph node involvement; the M category establishes presence of distance metastases. **Table 2** summarizes VIII edition of the TNM classification for lung cancer [13].

T	**Primary tumor**
TX	Primary tumor cannot be assessed or tumor proven by presence of malignant cells in sputum or bronchial washings but not visualized by imaging or bronchoscopy
T0	No evidence of primary tumor
Tis	Carcinoma *in situ*
T1	Tumor ≤3 cm in greatest dimension surrounded by lung or visceral pleura without bronchoscopic evidence of invasion more proximal than the lobar bronchus (i.e., not in the main bronchus)[1]
T1mi	Minimally invasive adenocarcinoma[2]
T1a	Tumor ≤1 cm in greatest dimension[1]
T1b	Tumor >1 cm but ≤2 cm in greatest dimension[1]
T1c	Tumor >2 cm but ≤3 cm in greatest dimension[1]
T2	Tumor >3 cm but ≤5 cm with any of the following features[3]: • Involving main bronchus regardless of distance from the carina, but without involving the carina • Invading visceral pleura • Presence of atelectasis or obstructive pneumonitis that extends to hilar region (involving part or entire lung)
T2a	Tumor >3 cm but ≤4 cm in greatest dimension
T2b	Tumor >4 cm but ≤5 cm in greatest dimension
T3	Tumor >5 cm but ≤7 cm in greatest dimension or direct invasion of chest wall (including superior sulcus tumor), phrenic nerve, parietal pericardium or separate tumor nodule(s) in the same lobe as the primary tumor
T4	Tumor >7 cm in greatest dimension or invasion of diaphragm, mediastinum, heart, great vessels, trachea, recurrent laryngeal nerve, esophagus, vertebral body, carina or separate nodule(s) in a different ipsilateral lobe to that of the primary tumor
N	Regional lymph nodes
NX	Regional lymph nodes cannot be assessed
N0	No regional lymph nodes metastasis
N1	Metastasis in ipsilateral peribronchial and/or ipsilateral hilar lymph nodes and intrapulmonary nodes, including involvement by direct extension
N2	Metastasis in ipsilateral mediastinal and7or subcarinal lymph node(s)
N3	Metastasis in contralateral mediastinal and hilar, ipsilateral or contralateral scalene or supraclavicular node(s)
M	Distant metastasis
M0	No distant metastasis
M1	Presence of distant metastasis
M1a	Separate tumor nodule(s) in a contralateral lobe to that of the primary tumor or tumor with pleural or pericardial nodule(s) or malignant pleural or pericardial effusion[4]
M1b	Single extrathoracic metastasis[5]
M1c	Multiple extrathoracic metastases to one or more organs

[1]*The uncommon superficial spreading tumor of any size with its invasive component limited to the bronchial wall, which may extend proximal to the main bronchus, is also classified as T1a.*

[2]*Solitary adenocarcinoma, ≤3 cm with a predominately lepidic pattern and ≤ 5 mm invasion in any 1 focus.*
[3]*T2 tumors with these features are classified as T2a if ≤4 cm in greatest dimension or if size cannot be determined, and T2b if >4 cm but ≤5 cm in greatest dimension.*
[4]*Most pleural/pericardial effusions with lung cancer are due to tumor. In a few patients, however, multiple microscopic examinations of pleural/pericardial fluid are negative for tumor. In these the effusion should be excluded as a staging descriptor.*
[5]*This includes involvement of a single distant (nonregional) lymph node.*

Table 2.
TNM classification.

In cases where CT does not show evidence of distant metastases, imaging staging should be completed with 18-FDG PET-CT, which has higher sensitivity and specificity than contrast-enhanced CT and higher sensitivity than (18)F-FDG PET in staging NSCLC in detecting extrathoracic and bone metastases. PET/TC has, however, low sensitivity in detecting brain metastases [14]. Staging brain MRI with contrast is used to evaluate the presence of cerebral metastases in patients with neurological symptoms or in the investigation of a suspected CT lesion [15].

Staging is divided into clinical staging (presurgical) and pathologic staging (after surgical resection of the tumor, lymph nodes or metastases) (**Table 3**).

4. Treatment of early stage lung cancer

Radical surgery allows to obtain a full recovery or to significantly improve the prognosis in patients with early stage disease and is not recommended for patients with advanced disease. Surgery needs to be taken in consideration in NSCLC stage I, II and in selected stage IIIA/IIIB (T1-T2, N2 single station, non-bulky). It should be performed in high-volume centers, by expert surgeons. It has been demonstrated that the outcome of patients undergoing lung resection for lung cancer is better for those treated in high-volume centers [16]. Before surgery, lung cancer patients need to be studied in order to define their operability. A tumor that can be completely resected with surgery is considered resectable. Even if a tumor is anatomically resectable, it is necessary to evaluate if the patient can tolerate surgery and is functionally operable according to his functional preoperative situation and, most importantly, his predicted postoperative status, especially with regard to respiratory and cardiovascular function. Cardiorespiratory evaluation is mandatory for patients that are candidate to a lung resection surgery, in order to predict the operatory risk and postoperative lung function. Lung function is evaluated mainly with: spirometry, Diffusion Lung CO (DLCO), hemogasanalysis, ergometric tests, lung perfusion scintigraphy. In case of lower values (FEV1 and DLCO <80%), Cardio Pulmonary Exercise Testing (CPET) is indicated and if the maximal oxygen consumption (VO2max) is less than 10 mL/kg/min the risk of serious postoperative complications is high. For cardiovascular assessment, the use of recalibrated thoracic Revised Cardiac Risk Index (RCRI) is recommended (**Table 4**).

An RCRI <2 has been reported to be associated with a low-cardiac risk, and no additional tests are needed. However, an RCRI >2 has been associated with an increased cardiac risk and a cardiac consultation with non-invasive testing is recommended [17, 18].

STAGE	T	N	M
Occult carcinoma	TX	N0	M0
0	Tis	N0	M0
IA1	T1mi	N0	M0
	T1a	N0	M0
IA2	T1b	N0	M0
IA3	T1c	N0	M0
IB	T2a	N0	M0
IIA	T2b	N0	M0
IIB	T1a	N1	M0
	T1b	N1	M0
	T1c	N1	M0
	T2a	N1	M0
	T2b	N1	M0
	T3	N0	M0
IIIA	T1a	N2	M0
	T1b	N2	M0
	T1c	N2	M0
	T2a	N2	M0
	T2b	N2	M0
	T3	N1	M0
	T4	N0	M0
	T4	N1	M0
IIIB	T1a	N3	M0
	T1b	N3	M0
	T1c	N3	M0
	T2a	N3	M0
	T2b	N3	M0
	T3	N2	M0
	T4	N2	M0
IIIC	T3	N3	M0
	T4	N3	Mo
IVA	Any T Any T	Any N Any N	M1a M1b
IVB	Any T	Any N	M1c

Table 3.
Staging of NSCLC.

Brunelli et al. [19] proposed a physiologic evaluation resection algorithm for major anatomic resection (lobectomy or greater).

For positive and low-risk or negative cardiac evaluation, we calculate postoperative FEV1 (ppoFEV1) and postoperative DLCO (ppoDLCO):

Weighted factors	Points
Ischaemic heart disease	1.5
History of cerebrovascular disease	1.5
Serum creatinine >2 mg/dL	1
Pneumonectomy planned	1.5
Classes of risk	
A	0
B	1–1.5
C	2–2.5
D	>2.5

Table 4.
Recalibrated thoracic revised cardiac risk index.

- If ppoFEV1 or ppoDLCO <30%, cardiopulmonary exercise test (CPET) is recommended.
    - If VO2max is >20 ml/kg/min or > 75%, the patient is considered at low risk for major anatomic resection.
    - If VO2max is 10–20 ml/kg/min or 35–75%, the patient is at moderate risk for major anatomic resection.
    - If VO2max is <10 ml/kg/min or < 35%, the patient is at high risk for major anatomic resection.
- If ppoFEV1 or ppoDLCO <60% and both >30%, stair climb or shuttle walk is recommended.
    - If stair climb is >22 m or shuttle walk is >400 m, the patient is considered at low risk for major anatomic resection.
    - If stair climb is <22 m or shuttle walk is <400 m, cardiopulmonary exercise test (CPET) is recommended.
- If ppoFEV1 and ppoDLCO is >60%, the patient is considered at low risk for major anatomic resection.

For positive high-risk cardiac evaluation, cardiopulmonary exercise test (CPET) is mandatory:

- If VO2max is >20 ml/kg/min or > 75%, the patient is considered at low risk for major anatomic resection.
- If VO2max is 10–20 ml/kg/min or 35–75%, the patient is at moderate risk for major anatomic resection.

- If VO2max is <10 ml/kg/min or < 35%, the patient is at high risk for major anatomic resection.

A multidisciplinary evaluation is necessary to discuss the different therapeutic options and their potential results. The surgical procedure depends on the extent and the localization of the tumor and on the cardiopulmonary reserve of the patients. Preoperative or intraoperative cytohistologic diagnosis is recommended before anatomic lobectomy, bilobectomy or pneumonectomy. Anyway, when the diagnosis is technically difficult to obtain, or it is at high risk for the patient and the radiological and clinical probability of lung cancer is high, it is possible to perform an anatomic resection without tissue confirmation of lung cancer.

Anatomic lobectomy with mediastinal lymphadenectomy is the gold standard treatment for lung cancer.

When the lesion is not resectable through a lobectomy, for instance if it infiltrates the main bronchus or the main artery, or if it invades the fissure to the adjacent lobe, pneumonectomy is indicated.

If anatomically applicable and if negative margin can be achieved, sleeve lobectomy is preferred over pneumonectomy.

Anatomic segmentectomy is acceptable for Ground Glass Opacities (GGO) or for very early stage of disease (Tis or T1a) or in patients who are not eligible for lobectomy. It is possible because GGO more often are diagnosed as in situ adenocarcinoma or minimally invasive adenocarcinoma. When segmentectomy is performed, parenchymal resection margins should be 2 cm or more, or they should be the size of the nodule or larger. In these cases, segmentectomy is preferred over wedge resection [20].

5. Surgical techniques

5.1 Thoracotomy

The first pulmonary resection for lung cancer was performed in 1912. At the beginning, surgical resection for lung cancer was pneumonectomy. In 1960s, lobectomy was recognized as the gold standard treatment. Traditional surgical approach was a 15–20 cm posterolateral thoracotomy. This traditional approach implies the resection of multiple muscle layers (latissimus dorsi and serratus anterior) and ribs divarication with metal retractors. Ribs fractures are common during divarication and sometimes ribs segments are resected to avoid fractures and to improve surgical exposure. This kind of thoracotomy allows an optimal view of the hilum and the use of two hands by the surgeon. This incision can result in pain and shoulder and chest wall dysfunction. 44% of patients undergoing thoracotomy develop chronic pain for 1 year after the procedure and 29% of patients experience pain for more than 1 year after surgery [21].

Noirclerc et al. [22] were the first to describe the muscle-sparing thoracotomy. The objective of this approach is to preserve muscles, in particular the latissimus dorsi. This technique reduces postoperative complications and consents a better postoperative mobilization of the shoulder, compared to traditional posterolateral thoracotomy.

5.2 Video-assisted thoracic surgery (VATS)

During the last decades, Minimally Invasive Surgery (MIS) was applied for lung cancer surgery. The first Video-Assisted Thoracoscopic Surgery (VATS) for lung resection was performed in the early 1990s [23]. At the beginning, the term VATS indicated the use of a videothoracoscope during thoracic surgery procedures, performed through traditional thoracotomy. For example, Okada et al. [24] described a hybrid approach, with a mini-thoracotomy and a camera port, used to see areas not visible with direct vision. Substantially, hybrid approach integrated direct and thoracoscopic vision. Then, there was the development of "pure" VATS using only thoracoscopic vision.

Most centers use a 3–5 cm utility incision located anteriorly, one port for the optic and another port located posteriorly. Gossot et al. [25] described pure thoracoscopic lobectomy using three incisions with a mini-thoracotomy for the extraction of the lobe. McKenna Jr. et al. [26] use three or occasionally four ports.

Hansen et al. [27] perform a standardized anterior three-port approach, with the ports located always in the same place, independently of the lobe to resect: a utility incision of 4–5 cm is located anteriorly at the 4th intercostal space, the 1–1,5 cm camera port is located anteriorly at the level of the diaphragm (8th intercostal space) and a posterior 1,5 cm incision is done at the same intercostal space.

Burfein and D'Amico perform double-port VATS lobectomy [28]: a 2 cm camera port is located at the 7th or 8th intercostal space in the mid-axillary line and a utility incision of 4,5 cm is located anteriorly at the 5th or 6th intercostal space. The double-port technique is characterized by a different lung exposure and the camera has to be moved between the camera port and the utility incision during surgery.

In all cases, systematic lymph node dissection is performed.

Compared to open approach, VATS lung resection is associated with lower postoperative pain, lower incidence of postoperative complications (including atrial fibrillation, atelectasis, prolonged air leak), shorter length of hospitalization, lower postoperative mortality. The reduced hospitalization also consents a rapid access to adjuvant chemotherapy [29]. Different studies analyzed the oncological equivalence of VATS compared to open approach. Some studies aimed to analyze the effectiveness of nodal dissection in VATS compared to that obtained with thoracotomy. Medbery et al. [30] affirmed that there is no difference in staging if nodal dissection is performed in high-volume centers. According to Watanabe et al. [31] a complete lymphadenectomy is possible in VATS also in N2 stage intraoperatively diagnosed. A retrospective study of the National Cancer Data Base (NCDB) showed no difference in nodal staging and overall survival between patients operated in VATS or in open resections [26]. It is also demonstrated that there is no difference in long-term survival [32].

During the years, VATS surgery evolved to a uniportal approach, with only a single incision used for all instruments and for lobe extraction. Rocco et al. [33] were the first to describe the uniportal approach in 2004 for wedge resection, not performing lobectomies. Gonzales-Rivas et al. [34] did the first uniportal VATS lobectomy in 2010. The utility incision is done at the 5th intercostal space, its size is the same of the utility incision used for triple or double-port approach. The surgeon and the assistant are placed both in front of the patient in order to have the same vision and to coordinate movements. A 30 degrees camera is used and it follows the instruments, giving a vision that closely resembles that of the open approach. Uniportal VATS lobectomy follows the same principles of all major pulmonary resection in VATS. Dissection of veins, arteries, bronchus and fissure is performed, with a complete mediastinal lymphadenectomy.

Different studies compared the outcome of uniportal and "multiportal" VATS, demonstrating a reduction of complications, length of hospitalization and duration of drain tube. Uniportal VATS also allows for a reduction in postoperative pain due to several factors. Firstly, it involves only one intercostal space, minimizing the overall surgical trauma. Secondly, the absence of trocars eliminates the potential compression on the intercostal nerve that may occur during the movements of the camera in traditional multiport VATS procedures [35]. An interesting evolution of the uniportal VATS was the development of the subxiphoid approach, in order to reduce the pain due to intercostal nerve damage [36]. It also can be used to treat bilateral disease, even if the visualization is limited, compared to transthoracic techniques [37]. More studies are necessary to compare subxiphoid to transthoracic approach.

General anesthesia with single lung ventilation is required for lung surgery and it is obtained through a double lumen endotracheal tube or through a bronchial blocker. The patient is positioned in lateral position. Both the surgeon and the assistant stay in front of the patient in order to have the same vision. In general, the port position is the same for every lobectomy. A 30° videothoracoscope and long and curved instruments are usually used. Hilum dissection is performed bluntly with instruments, suction device, peanuts or energy devices. Vascular and bronchial elements are isolated and resected through linear endo-staplers. Also the fissure is divided with endo-stapler device. The specimen is extracted using an endo-bag. The chest tube is inserted in the camera port at the end of surgery. Then, the lymphadenectomy is done mainly using energy device.

Lymphadenectomy is necessary for the correct staging of the disease. Systematic lymph node dissection is recommended. Anyway some authors recommend the lobe-specific mediastinal lymphadenectomy. According to them, nodal metastasis is related to the localization of the primary tumor: upper lobe tumors tend to metastasize upper lymph nodes and lower lobe tumors tend to spread to the inferior and subcarinal nodes [38]. Systematic mediastinal lymph node dissection allows the detection of more metastatic lymph nodes and a better oncologic outcome than lobe-specific nodal dissection [39]. Gooseman and Brunelli [40] recommend systematic lymphadenectomy and in particular, even for the selected cases in which lobe-specific nodal dissection could be accepted (peripheral T1 squamous cell carcinoma), they recommend always the dissection of subcarinal lymph nodes.

The surgeon has to be prepared to convert to thoracotomy in case of technical difficulties in dissection or in case of bleeding.

5.2.1 Right upper lobectomy

The first step involves performing a mediastinal release maneuver. The lung is retracted anteriorly and the posterior pleura is dissected at the level of the bronchial bifurcation. It helps the dissection of the bronchus from the anterior approach. Then, the lung is retracted posteriorly and the dissection of the veins is performed. Once identified and dissected the upper lobe vein, it is resected with vascular endo-stapler. The resection of the vein exposes the pulmonary artery. The arterial branches to the upper lobe (truncus anterior and ascending arteries) are dissected and divided through vascular endo-stapler. Then, the bronchus is divided through bronchial stapler and the fissure is completed with endo-stapler device. The specimen is extracted in an endo-bag through the utility incision.

5.2.2 Left upper lobectomy

The lung is retracted anteriorly and the posterior pleura is dissected in order to identify the posterior artery and to facilitate the maneuvers with the anterior approach. The lung is retracted posteriorly and, after the identification of the veins, the upper lobe vein is dissected and divided through endo-stapler, exposing the pulmonary artery and the upper lobe bronchus. The arterial branches for the anterior, posterior and apical segments and the lingular branches are exposed and divided through vascular endo-staplers. Then, the upper bronchus and the major fissure are divided through endo-staplers. The specimen is extracted in an endo-bag through the utility incision.

5.2.3 Middle lobectomy

The middle lobe vein is dissected and divided. Then the fissure to the lower lobe and the bronchus to the middle lobe are divided through endo-staplers. Then the artery branches are dissected and divided and at the end the fissure to the upper lobe is completed through endo-stapler. The specimen is extracted in an endo-bag through the utility incision.

5.2.4 Lower lobectomies

The first step of lower lobectomies is represented by the division of the inferior pulmonary ligament. This confers mobility to the lobe and exposes the vein to the lower lobe. The lower lobe vein is dissected and divided with endo-stapler (**Figure 2**). Then the procedure can continue in two ways: the surgeon can dissect the arterial branches to the lower lobe (for the apical segment and for the basal pyramid) and the bronchus to the lower lobe within the fissure. The other option is represented by the fissureless technique: after the dissection and resection of the vein, the lower lobe is retracted cranially and the plane between the bronchus and the artery is dissected and

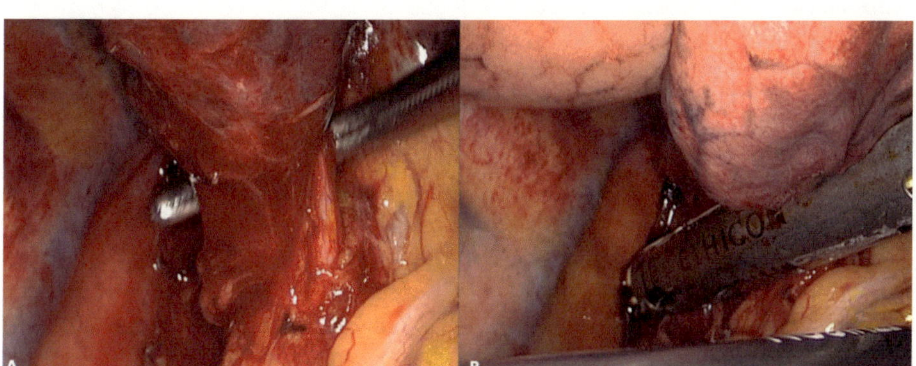

Figure 2.
Right lower lobectomy: (A) right lower lobe vein dissection; (B) right lower lobe division through endo-stapler.

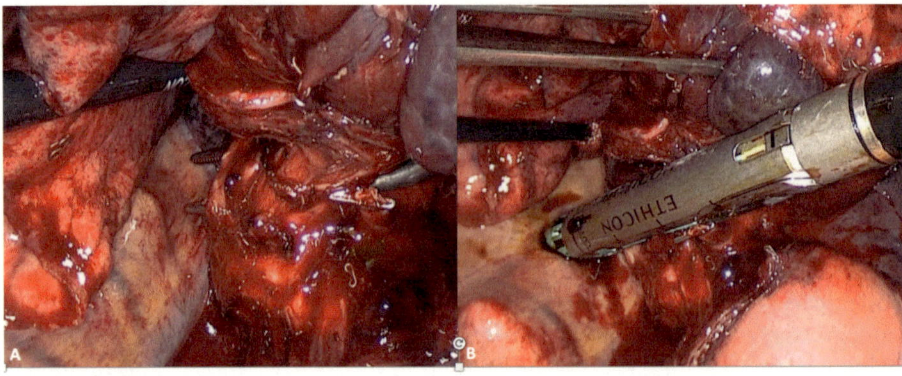

Figure 3.
Right lower lobectomy: (A) dissection right lower lobe bronchus; (B) division of right of right lower lobe bronchus through endo-stapler.

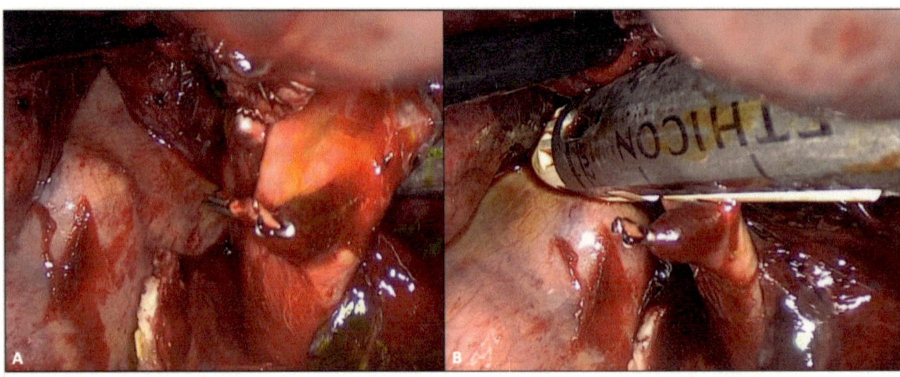

Figure 4.
Right lower lobe artery: (A) dissection and (B) division of right lower lobe artery through endo-stapler.

the bronchus is divided through endo-stapler (**Figure 3**). Then, the arterial branches are divided and the fissure is divided at last (**Figure 4**). The specimen is extracted in an endo-bag through the utility incision.

5.3 Robotic-assisted thoracic surgery (RATS)

The most recent minimally invasive technique applied to thoracic surgery is robotic approach. The progress in the field of robotic technology generated interest in thoracic surgeons, that started to perform Robot-Assisted Thoracic Surgery (RATS). The first robotic lobectomies were described by Morgan et al. [41] and by Ashton et al. [42] in 2003. Since then, robotic lobectomy started to be performed in different centers. Cerfolio et al. [43] described their initial results using a completely portal 4-arm robotic operation with insufflation of carbon dioxide. The four ports are located at the same intercostal space (7th intercostal space). They achieved a complete R0 resection, performing a median number of 5 mediastinal lymph node station dissections. They recorded a significant reduction in morbidity and hospital stay compared to thoracotomy. When compared to VATS, Kent et al. [44] reported less postoperative pain and a rapid return to normal activities.

In 2021, Yang et al. [45] were the first to describe a uniportal RATS lobectomy for a tumor located in the right upper lobe. A single 4 cm incision was made at the 4th intercostal space on the mid-axillary line. The 30° camera arm was placed on the upper end of the incision and the two instrument arms were placed intercrossed inside the chest. With this approach, they were able to perform a radical lobectomy and lymphadenectomy. The recovery was fast and the patient was discharged three days after surgery.

RATS consents a three-dimensional (3D) high-definition view, intuitive articulation of the robotic hands and more flexibility of instruments, with seven degrees of motion. Its superior instrumentations consent to perform accurate and safe dissection, in particular lymph node dissection that is crucial for the correct staging of lung cancer. It also can be used for difficult cases at high risk of conversion such as central tumors, sleeve lobectomy and pneumonectomy. To date, studies comparing VATS and RATS lobectomy do not show significant differences in terms of outcome. For this reason, a challenging question arises regarding the cost-benefit analysis [46, 47].

6. Conclusions and future perspectives

At the beginning of the era of minimally invasive thoracic surgery, a great limit of the technique was represented by the vision, because of the low definitions of cameras. Surgeons preferred the direct vision to have a better control of the procedure. The progress in the field of technologies consented to have high-definition cameras also with additional features, such as 3d vision or integration with augmented reality surgery navigation systems. Nowadays, cameras are largely used by surgeons even in thoracotomy approach to improve visualization and lightning. The progress made in the field of instrumentations has been appreciated by surgeons and instruments made for minimally invasive surgery such as endo-staplers are now used also for open approach, because of their thickness and flexibility.

Another challenge for VATS surgery is the use of rigid instruments that have to be moved through the rigid chest wall. Human hand consents to perform several traction and counter-traction movement and provides tactile feedback. With the development of minimally invasive surgery, that limits the tactile feedback, surgeons started to operate mainly relying on the vision. This happens, in particular, in RATS. Since the chance to palpate nodules or ground glass opacities is little in VATS and even null in RATS, surgeons has to rely only on visual signals. For this reason, they can use intraoperative ultrasound or they can mark nodules with coils in hybrid operating room [48]. Also artificial intelligence is developing in order to help surgeons during procedures.

The field of minimally invasive thoracic surgery is developing in two directions: reducing the number and the size of the surgical access (uniportal VATS) and increasing the use of RATS. The objective is to combine the advantage of uniportal VATS (lower postoperative pain, enhanced recovery) and RATS (better visualization, more degrees of movements).

Author details

Gaetana Messina[1*], Mary Bove[1], Giorgia Opromolla[1], Vincenzo Di Filippo[1], Mario Pirozzi[2], Marianna Caterino[2], Sergio Facchini[2], Alessia Zotta[2], Giovanni Vicidomini[1], Mario Santini[1], Alfonso Fiorelli[1], Fortunato Ciardiello[2] and Morena Fasano[2]

1 Thoracic Surgery Unit, Università degli Studi della Campania "Luigi Vanvitelli", Napoli, Campania, Italy

2 Department of Precision Medicine, Università della Campania "L. Vanvitelli", Napoli, Campania, Italy

*Address all correspondence to: adamessina@virgilio.it

References

[1] Siegel RL, Miller KD, Fuchs HE, Jemal A. Cancer statistics, 2022. CA: A Cancer Journal for Clinicians. 2022;**72**:7-33

[2] Howlader N. SEER Cancer Statistics Review, 1975-2018, based on November 2020 SEER data submission, Bethesda, MD: National Cancer Institute, April 2021. [Online]. Available from: https://seer.cancer.gov/csr/1975_2018/

[3] Alberg AJ, Brock MV, Samet JM. Epidemiology of lung cancer: Looking to the future. Journal of Clinical Oncology. 2005;**23**(31):75-85

[4] Bethune G, Bethune D, Ridgway N, Xu Z. Epidermal growth factor receptor (EGFR) in lung cancer: An overview and update. Journal of Thoracic Disease. 2010;**2**(1):48-51

[5] National Lung Screening Trial Research Team, Aberle DR, Berg CD, Black WC, Church TR, Fagerstrom RM, et al. The National Lung Screening Trial: Overview and study design. Radiology. 2011;**258**:243-253

[6] Nicholson AG, Tsao MS, Beasley MB, Borczuk AC, Brambilla E, Cooper WA, et al. The 2021 WHO classification of lung tumors: Impact of advances since 2015. Journal of Thoracic Oncology. 2022;**17**(3):362-387

[7] Forde PM, Ettinger DS. Targeted therapy for non-small-cell lung cancer: Past, present and future. Expert Review of Anticancer Therapy. 2013;**13**:745-758

[8] Walling AM, Weeks JC, Kahn KL, Tisnado D, Keating NL, Dy SM, et al. Symptom prevalence in lung and Colo-rectal cancer patients. Journal of Pain and Symptom Management. 2015;**49**(2):192-202

[9] Panunzio A, Sartori P. Lung cancer and radiological imaging. Current Radiopharmaceuticals. 2020;**13**(3):238-242

[10] Vlahos I, Stefanidis K, Sheard S, Nair A, Sayer C, Moser J. Lung cancer screening: Nodule identification and characterization. Translational Lung Cancer Research. 2018;**7**(3):288-303

[11] Chao F, Zhang H. PET/CT in the staging of the non-small cell lung cancer. Journal of Biomedicine & Biotechnology. 2012;**2012**:783739

[12] Remon J, Soria J-C, Peters S. ESMO guidelines committee. Early and locally advanced non-small cell lung cancer (NSCLC): ESMO clinical practice guidelines for diagnosis, treatment and follow-up. Annals of Oncology. 2017;**28**(4):iv1-iv21

[13] Network NCC. Non-small cell lung cancer (version 3.2022), NCCN clinical practice guidelines in oncology. Journal of the National Comprehensive Cancer Network. 2022;**20**(5):497-530

[14] Wu Y, Li P, Zhang H, Shi Y, Wu H, Zhang J, et al. Diagnostic value of fluorine 18 fluorodeoxyglucose positron emission tomography/computed tomography for the detection of metastases in non-small-cell lung cancer patients. International Journal of Cancer. 2013;**132**(2):E37-E47

[15] Kim M, Suh CH, Lee SM, Kim HC, Aizer AA, Yanagihara TK, et al. Diagnostic yield of staging brain MRI in patients with newly diagnosed non-small cell lung cancer. Radiology. 2020;**297**(2):419-427

[16] Rea F, Ieva F, Pastorino U, Apolone G, Barni S, Merlino L, et al. Number of lung resections performed and long-term mortality rates of patients after lung cancer surgery: Evidence from an Italian investigation. European Journal of Cardio-Thoracic Surgery. 2020;**58**(1):70-77

[17] Brunelli A, Varela G, Salati M, Jimenez MF, Pompili C, Novoa N, et al. Recalibration of the revised cardiac risk index in lung resection candidates. The Annals of Thoracic Surgery. 2010;**90**(1):199-203

[18] Brunelli A, Cassivi SD, Fibla J, Halgren LA, Wigle DA, Allen MS, et al. External validation of the recalibrated thoracic revised cardiac risk index for predicting the risk of major cardiac complications after lung resection. The Annals of Thoracic Surgery. 2011;**92**(2):445-448

[19] Brunelli A, Kim AW, Berger KI, Addrizzo-Harris DJ. Physiologic evaluation of the patient with lung cancer being considered for resectional surgery: Diagnosis and management of lung cancer. Chest. 2013;**143**(5 Suppl.):e166S-e190S

[20] Jiang L, Yin W, Peng G, Wang W, Zhang J, Liu Y, et al. Prognosis and status of lymph node involvement in patients with adenocarcinoma in situ and minimally invasive adenocarcinoma-a systematic literature review and pooled-data analysis. Journal of Thoracic Disease. 2015;**7**:2003-2009

[21] Landreneau RJ, Mack MJ, Hazelrigg SR, Naunheim K, Dowling RD, Ritter P, et al. Prevalence of chronic pain after pulmonary resection by thoracotomy or video-assisted thoracic surgery. The Journal of Thoracic and Cardiovascular Surgery. 1994;**107**(4):1079-1085

[22] Noirclerc M, Dor V, Chauvin G, Kreitman P, Masselot R, Balenbois D, et al. Extensive lateral thoracotomy without muscle section. Annales de Chirurgie Thoracique et Cardio-Vasculaire. 1973;**12**:181-184

[23] Hazelrigg SR, Nunchuck SK, LoCicero J 3rd. Hazelrigg SR, video assisted thoracic surgery study group data. The Annals of Thoracic Surgery. 1993;**56**:1039-1043

[24] Okada M, Sakamoto T, Yuki T, Mimura T, Miyoshi K, Tsubota N. Hybrid surgical approach of video-assisted minithoracotomy for lung cancer: Significance of direct visualization on quality of surgery. Chest. 2005;**128**(4):2696-2701

[25] Gossot D, Girard P, Raynaud C, Stern J-B, Caliandro R, Validire P, et al. Totally endoscopic major pulmonary resection for stage I bronchial carcinoma: Initial results. Revue des Maladies Respiratoires. 2009;**26**(9):961-970

[26] McKenna R, J Jr, Houck W, Fuller CB. Video-assisted thoracic surgery lobectomy: Experience with 1,100 cases. Annals of Thoracic Surgery. 2006;**81**(2):421-425

[27] Hansen HJ, Petersen RH, Christensen M. Video-assisted thoracoscopic surgery (VATS) lobectomy using a standardized anterior approach. Surgical Endoscopy. 2011;**25**(4):1263-1269

[28] Burfeind WR, D'Amico TA. Thoracoscopic lobectomy. Operative Techniques in Thoracic and Cardiovascular Surgery. 2004;**9**(2):98-114

[29] Petersen RP, Pham DK, Burfeind WR, Hanish SI, Toloza EM, Harpole DH Jr, et al. Thoracoscopic

lobectomy facilitates the delivery of chemotherapy after resection for lung cancer. Annals of Thoracic Surgery. 2007;**83**(4):1245-1250

[30] Medbery RL, Gillespie TW, Liu Y, Nickleach DC, Lipscomb J, Sancheti MS, et al. Nodal upstaging is more common with thoracotomy than with vats during lobectomy for early-stage lung cancer: An analysis from the national cancer data base. Journal of Thoracic Oncology. 2016;**11**(2):222-233

[31] Watanabe A, Mishina T, Ohori S, Koyanagi T, Nakashima S, Mawatari T, et al. Is video-assisted thoracoscopic surgery a feasible approach for clinical N0 and postoperatively pathological N2 non-small cell lung cancer? European Journal of Cardio-Thoracic Surgery. 2008;**33**(5):812-818

[32] Flores RM, Park BJ, Dycoco J, Aronova A, Hirth Y, Rizk NP, et al. Lobectomy by video-assisted thoracic surgery (VATS) versus thoracotomy for lung cancer. The Journal of Thoracic and Cardiovascular Surgery. 2009;**138**(1):11-18

[33] Rocco G, Martin-Ucar A, Passera E. Uniportal VATS wedge pulmonary resections. Annals of Thoracic Surgery. 2004;**77**(2):726-728

[34] Gonzalez D, Paradela M, Garcia J, Dela Torre M. Single-port video-assisted thoracoscopic lobectomy. Interactive Cardiovascular and Thoracic Surgery. 2011;**12**(3):514-516

[35] Harris CG, James RS, Tian DH, Yan TD, Doyle MP, Gonzalez-Rivas D, et al. Systematic review and meta-analysis of uniportal versus multiportal video-assisted thoracoscopic lobectomy for lung cancer. The Annals of Cardiothoracic Surgery. 2016;**5**(2):76-84

[36] Liu C-C, Wang B-Y, Shih C-S, Liu Y-H. Subxiphoid single-incision thoracoscopic left upper lobectomy. The Journal of Thoracic and Cardiovascular Surgery. 2014;**148**(6):3260-3251

[37] Gonzalez-Rivas D, Lirio F, Sesma J, Akar FA. Subxiphoid complex uni- portal video-assisted major pulmonary resections. The Journal of Visualized Surgery. 2017;**3**:93

[38] Aokage K, Yoshida J, Ishii G, Hishida T, Nishimura M, Nagai K. Subcarinal lymph node in upper lobe non-small cell lung cancer patients: Is selective lymph node dissection valid? Lung Cancer. 2017;**70**(2):163-167

[39] Handa Y, Tsutani Y, Mimae T, Miyata Y, Ito H, Shimada Y, et al. Systematic versus lobe-specific mediastinal lymphadenectomy for Hypermetabolic lung cancer. Annals of Surgical Oncology. 2021;**28**:7162-7171

[40] Gooseman MBA. Intraoperative lymph node management during non-small cell lung cancer surgery. Annals of Surgical Oncology. 2021;**28**:6925-6926

[41] Morgan JA, Ginsburg ME, Sonett JR, Morales DLS, Kohmoto T, Gorenstein LA, et al. Advanced thoracoscopic procedures are facilitated by computer-aided robotic technology. European Journal of Cardio-Thoracic Surgery. 2003;**23**:883-887

[42] Ashton RC Jr, Connery CP, Swistel DG, DeRose JJ Jr. Robot-assisted lobectomy. The Journal of Thoracic and Cardiovascular Surgery. 2003;**126**:292-293

[43] Cerfolio RJ, Bryant AS, Skylizard L, Minnich DJ. Initial consecutive experience of completely portal robotic pulmonary resection with 4 arms. The Journal of Thoracic and Cardiovascular Surgery. 2011;**142**(4):740-746

[44] Kent M, Wang T, Whyte R, Curran T, Flores R, Gangadharan S. Open, video-assisted thoracic surgery, and robotic lobectomy: Review of a national database. The Annals of Thoracic Surgery. 2014;**97**(1):236-242

[45] Yang Y, Song L, Huang J, Cheng X, Luo Q. A uniportal right upper lobectomy by three-arm robotic-assisted thoracoscopic surgery using the da Vinci (xi) surgical system in the treatment of early-stage lung cancer. Translational Lung Cancer Research. 2021;**10**(3):1571-1575

[46] Swanson SJ, Miller DL, Robert Joseph McKenna JH Jr, Marshall MB, Yoo AC, Moore M, et al. Comparing robot-assisted thoracic surgical lobectomy with conventional video-assisted thoracic surgical lobectomy and wedge resection: Results from a multihospital database (premier). The Journal of Thoracic and Cardiovascular Surgery. 2014;**147**(3):929-937

[47] Gómez-Hernández MT, Fuentes MG, Novoa NM, Rodríguez I, Varela G, Jiménez MF. Similar outcomes after newly implemented rats approach compared to standard vats for anatomical lung resection. A propensity-score matched analysis. Cir Esp (Engl Ed). Aug 2022;**100**(8):504-510

[48] Ujiie H, Kato T, Hu H-P, Patel P, Wada H, Fujino K, et al. A novel minimally invasive near-infrared thoracoscopic localization technique of small pul- monary nodules: A phase I feasibility trial. The Journal of Thoracic and Cardiovascular Surgery. 2017;**154**(2):702-711

Chapter 3

Trends of Pediatric Cancer in India

Sajna Panolan, Srinivas Govindarajulu, S. Kalpana, Valarmathi Srinivasan and Joseph Maria Adaikalam

Abstract

Compared to developed countries, only a limited number of studies systematically engage with India's experience with the burden of childhood cancer and its implications for public healthcare in the country. This study aims to assess the long-term trend in the incidence of cancerous conditions, demographic factors, and the burden of the disease among children. The study has used the Madras Metropolitan Tumor Registry (MMTR), covering cancer cases reported among children (0–14 years) in Chennai for the last 34 years (1982–2016). The study analyses the incidence of the pediatric tumor for different age groups, gender, and type of cancer and the long-term trend over the years and compares the same with existing studies. The trend indicates that more cases are reported during 2007-11and the least number of cases are reported during 2012–2016 (respectively 16.7% and 11.9% of total cases reported).

Keywords: childhood cancer, pediatric cancer, tumor, trend, Chennai

1. Introduction

Globally, the incidence of childhood cancer has been increasing steadily and throws new challenges in public health management and policy making. Its nature, types and risk factors vary across the countries. As a developing country, India's experience with its given context is very important in understanding the role of epidemiological, demographic, socio-economic factors, and policy engagements in addressing public healthcare challenges. Several studies are looking into the experience of developed countries in addressing the cancer prevalence of cancer among children, their treatment, and attempts to connect them with countries' epidemiological transition. Compared to this, only a limited number of studies systematically engage with India's experience with the burden of childhood cancer and its implications for public healthcare in the country.

Available evidence indicates that India also experiences a steady increase in the number of children affected by different types of cancer. The details suggest that leukemia is the most common cancer affecting children followed by lymphoma and retinoblastoma. The profile of children affected by cancer shows variation across the age groups. The incidence of retinoblastoma, renal tumors, neuroblastoma, and hepatic tumors was found higher among children aged below five years whereas lymphoma, leukemia, bone tumors, and central nervous system tumors were found more among children aged above five years [1].

Globally, the annual number of new cases of childhood cancer exceeds 2, 00,000 and more than 80 percent of the reported cases are from the developing world [2]. Thirteen percent of the annual deaths worldwide are cancer-related and 70 percent of them are in the low- and middle-income countries [3]. Childhood cancer (age at diagnosis 0–14 years) is associated with a variety of malignancies and its incidence varies by age, sex, ethnicity, and geography, as reported by canceretiology [4, 5]. The incidence of childhood cancer across the countries ranges from 75 to 150 per million children per year. For instance, only 0.5 percent of all cancer cases reported in England occur in children less than 15 years of age whereas in India this proportion appears higher at 1.6–4.8 percent with variation by place of residence. This is related to the population structure (33% of the population in India is less than 15 years of age compared to 18% in England) [6, 7]. Though it remains less than the cases reported in the developed world, about 1.6 to 4.8 percent of all cancer reported in India are found in children below 15 years of age, and the overall incidence of 38 to 124 per million children, per year [8].

As 75 percent of the world population lives in these countries, developing countries bear more than half of the global cancer burden [9]. Because of population growth, aging and urbanization, changing dietary habits, better control of infections, and increasing tobacco consumption, developing countries are anticipated to bear a greater cancer burden, including that of greater lympho-hemopoietic malignancies [10]. India found to have 3 million persons is reported with cancer at any time, with 0.8 million new cases of cancer diagnosed each year [11]. There is a constant rise in cancer cases, but the trend and pattern vary according to the geographical region [12].

India's experience with a fast-growing economy and change in lifestyle-related behaviors can be connected to increasing cancer load [13, 14]. The relative differences in the incidence of lympho-hemopoietic malignancies in urban and rural populations can be connected with the differences in the environmental and socioeconomic factors affecting the dietary habits and lifestyle in rural and urban areas [15]. They tend to follow the larger trends noticed in terms of disease risk connected with the relative contributions of environment and genetics in the etiology of specific cancers. Studies consider their contribution to risk due to variation in exposure to carcinogens (in the external environment, or through lifestyle choices), or in genetic susceptibility to them [16].

This study broadly highlights the intensity of childhood cancer and its implications for child healthcare and health management in the global, national and local contexts. It aims to assess the long-term trend in the incidence of cancerous conditions, demographic factors, and the burden of the disease among children in Chennai from 1982 to 2016.

2. Materials and methods

This study has used the Madras Metropolitan Tumor Registry (MMTR), a population-based cancer registry (PBCR) based at the Cancer Institute (WIA), Chennai covering all cases reported among children (0–14 years) in Chennai for the last 34 years (1982–2016). All cases of childhood cancer from 0 to 14 years of age that were registered from 1st January 1982 to 31st December 2016 were included in this study. The study analyses the data on the incidence of the pediatric tumor for different age group, gender, and type of cancer and the long-term trend over the years and compare the same with existing studies. Childhood cancers (age at diagnosis

0–14 years) comprise a variety of malignancies, with incidence varied by age, sex, and ethnicity that provided insights into cancer etiology. The analysis looks into the types and incidence rate of cancer across the different age groups of children. The proposal was reviewed and approved by the ethical and scientific committees of the university.

3. Result and discussion

The analysis covers 34 years (1982 and 2016) and shows the trend of the cancerous condition of children of madras. The long-term trend indicates that more number of cases is reported during 2007–2011 (639cases) constitutes 16.7 percent of the total cases reported during this period. At the same time, the least number of cases are reported during 2012–2016 (458cases), constituting 11.9 percent of the total cases reported (**Figure 1**).

Table 1 describes the Sex-wise distribution of pediatric cancer during this period and shows that more number of cases are reported among male children (2313 cases) constituting 60.3% of total cases reported (3834). Compared to this, only 1521 cases (39.7%) are reported among female children.

Figure 2 describes the age group distribution of pediatric cancer reported from 1982 to 2016. When the children are classified into three agegroups, the data shows that more pediatric cancer is reported in 0–4 years of age (1417 cases) accounting for 37 percent of the total cases reported (3834 cases). The details show that the highest number of cases (370 cases, constituting 9.7%) was reported at three years of age.

Table 2 shows the distribution of reported cases among the major religious groups. Compared to other religious groups, more pediatric cancer cases were reported in the Hindu community, (3172 cases) constituting 82.7 percent of the total 3834 cases. A large number of cases were reported among children from Muslim (392 cases, 10.2%), and Christian (247 cases 6.4%) communities.

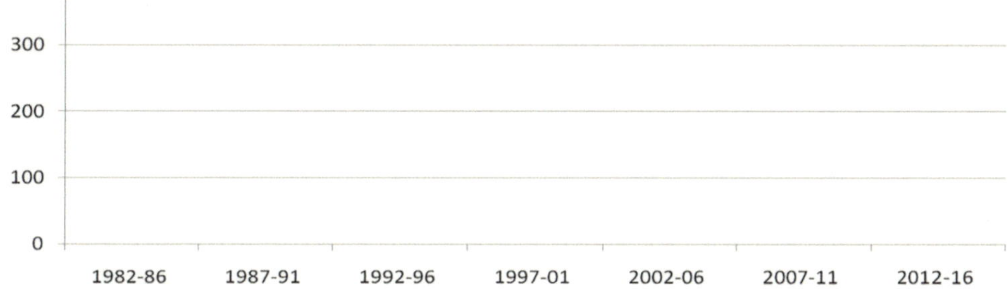

Figure 1.
Number of cases reported: 1982–2016.

SEX	Frequency	Percent (%)
Male	2313	60.3
Female	1521	39.7
Total	3834	100

Table 1.
Sex-wise distribution of reported cases (1982–2016).

Religion	Frequency	Percent (%)
Hindu	3172	82.7
Muslim	392	10.2
Christian	247	6.4
Sikh	1	0.0
Jain	22	0.6
Total	3834	100

Table 2.
Religion-wise distribution of reported cases 1982–2016.

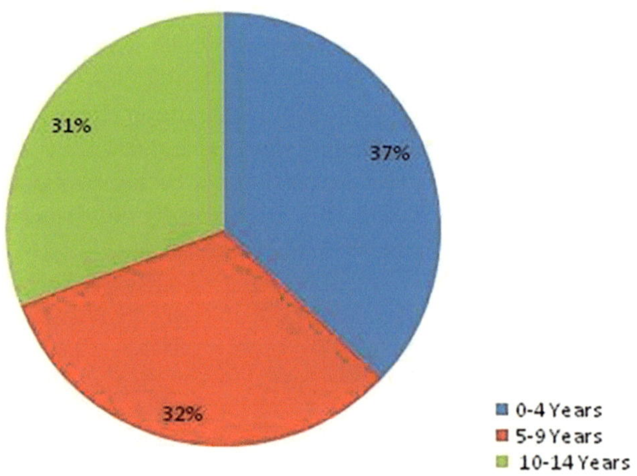

Figure 2.
Distribution of reported cases across the age groups (share in %).

Table 3 describes the distribution of different types of pediatric cancer reported during this period. The trend indicates that lymphoid leukemia is the most common type of cancer reported (1002 cases, constituting 26.1% of 3834 cases). Non-Hodgkin's lymphoma, Myeloid Leukemia, Hodgkin's disease, Brain Tumor, Eye Cancer, and other type's cancers.

Table 4 shows that the pattern of reported cases changes across the years. Types of major cancer reported between different periods show that more number of cases were reported during 2007–2011 (639 cases, 16.7%). Major types include Non-Hodgkin's lymphoma (39 cases, 6.1%), brain tumor (29 cases, 4.5%), rectum cancer

Type of CA	Frequency	Percent (%)
Lymphoid Leukemia	1002	26.1
NHL	297	7.7
Myeloid Leukemia	261	6.8
Hodgkin's Disease	204	5.3
Brain Tumor	139	3.6
Eye Cancer	120	3.1
Other Cancer	1124	29.3
Bone Cancer	95	2.5
Rectum Cancer	192	5.0
Testis Cancer	53	1.4
Adrenal gland Cancer	69	1.8
Liver Cancer	40	1.0
Kidney Cancer	140	3.7
Leukemia unspecific	46	1.2
Multiple myeloma	52	1.4
Total	3834	100

Table 3.
Major types of cancer reported 1982–2016.

(37 cases, 5.8%), kidney cancer (33cases, 5.2%), and other cancers (219cases, 34.3%). The other categories of cancer include cancers of the Nose, Pinna, fingers, nasopharyngeal cancers, etc.

Figure 3 shows the distribution of reported cases with their types and gender. The trend indicates that most types of cancer reported remain high among the male children, except myeloid leukemia (7.1%), eye cancer (4%), bone cancer (2.7%), liver cancer (1.2%), kidney cancer (4.1%) and other types of cancers (33.9%).

Table 5 shows the incidence of different types of pediatric cancer for different age groups. More pediatric cancers are reported in 0–4 years of age (1417 cases, 37%) out of 3834cases. Which include myeloid leukemia (14.7%), eye cancer (6.4%), adrenal gland cancer (3.8%), liver cancer (2.3%), and multiple myeloma (1.5%). Compared to this, more cases of lymphoid leukemia (29.1%), non-Hodgkin's lymphoma (9%), Hodgkin's disease (7%), brain tumor (5.2%), rectum cancer (5.1%), testis cancer (2.3%), kidney cancer (4.2%), and unspecific leukemia (1.3%) were reported in 5–9 years of age. The number of cases reported on Bone cancer (2.5%), and other cancer (29.3%) was found high among the children 10–14 years of age.

The overall incidence of pediatric cancer has gradually decreased in Chennai during the period 2012–2016, compared to the previous years. Leukemia emerges as the most common pediatric cancer as indicated by many studies (**Table 4**). The results broadly follow some of the existing studies like the highest incidence occurring between 0 and 4 years of age (**Table 2**) and non-Hodgkin's disease exceeds Hodgkin's disease (**Table 4**) as reported in India between 2012 and 2014 (Suman

Types	1982–1986	1987–1991	1992–1996	1997–2001	2002–2006	2007–2011	2012–2016	Total
Lymphoid Leukemia	92 (19.4)	106 (21.7)	173 (28.7)	138 (25.5)	209 (33.2)	172 (26.9)	112 (24.5)	1002 (26.1)
NHL	51 (10.7)	43 (8.8)	57 (9.5)	48 (8.9)	34 (5.4)	39 (6.1)	25 (5.5)	297 (7.7)
Myeloid Leukemia	44 (9.3)	50 (10.2)	34 (5.6)	32 (5.9)	41 (6.5)	31 (4.9)	29 (6.3)	261 (6.8)
Hodgkin's D	19 (4.0)	38 (7.8)	35 (5.8)	35 (6.5)	31 (4.9)	26 (4.1)	20 (4.4)	204 (5.3)
Brain Tumor	14 (2.9)	30 (6.1)	14 (2.3)	13 (2.4)	22 (3.5)	29 (4.5)	17 (3.7)	139 (3.6)
Eye Cancer	29 (6.1)	18 (3.7)	26 (4.3)	39 (7.2)	8 (1.3)	0 (0.0)	0 (0.0)	120 (3.1)
Other CA	147 (30.9)	138 (28.3)	165 (27.4)	136 (25.1)	164 (26.0)	219 (34.3)	155 (33.8)	1124 (29.3)
Bone CA	13 (2.7)	16 (3.3)	13 (2.2)	13 (2.4)	16 (2.5)	10 (1.6)	14 (3.1)	95 (2.5)
Rectum CA	24 (5.1)	23 (4.7)	31 (5.1)	24 (4.4)	28 (4.4)	37 (5.8)	25 (5.5)	192 (5.0)
Testis CA	11 (2.3)	8 (1.6)	12 (2.0)	8 (1.5)	9 (1.4)	2 (0.3)	3 (0.7)	53 (1.4)
Adrenal gland CA	3 (0.6)	0 (0.0)	0 (0.0)	8 (1.5)	18 (2.9)	18 (2.8)	22 (4.8)	69 (1.8)
Liver CA	3 (0.6)	2 (0.4)	11 (1.8)	3 (0.6)	8 (1.3)	7 (1.1)	6 (1.3)	40 (1.0)
Kidney CA	14 (2.9)	10 (2.0)	14 (2.3)	22 (4.1)	27 (4.3)	33 (5.2)	20 (4.4)	140 (3.7)
Leukemia unspecific	3 (0.6)	4 (0.8)	8 (1.3)	14 (2.6)	9 (1.4)	5 (0.8)	3 (0.7)	46 (1.2)
Multiple myeloma	8 (1.7)	2 (0.4)	9 (1.5)	9 (1.7)	6 (1.0)	11 (1.7)	7 (1.5)	52 (1.4)
Total	475 (100)	488 (100)	602 (100)	542 (100)	630 (100)	639 (100)	458 (100)	3834 (100)

Table 4.
Major types of cancer: Trends across specific intervals (share in %).

Das et. al) [17]. Similarly, overall cancer in children is more common among males than females (Stiller C 2007; [18] Gurney JG. et al. 2006) [19]. Existing studies report that both Hodgkin's and Non-Hodgkin's disease had the highest incidence among 10–14 years age group for both sexes (Suman Das.et al. 2017) whereas the present study finds that the Non-Hodgkin's disease and Hodgkin's disease had the highest incidence among 5–9 years of age group (**Table 5**). Our analysis also highlights that brain tumor had the highest incidence among 5–9 years of the age group for both sexes (**Table 5**). Eye and liver tumors had the highest incidence among the 0–4 years age group while bone and gastrointestinal tumors had the highest incidence among the 10–14 years age group for both sexes (**Table 5**).

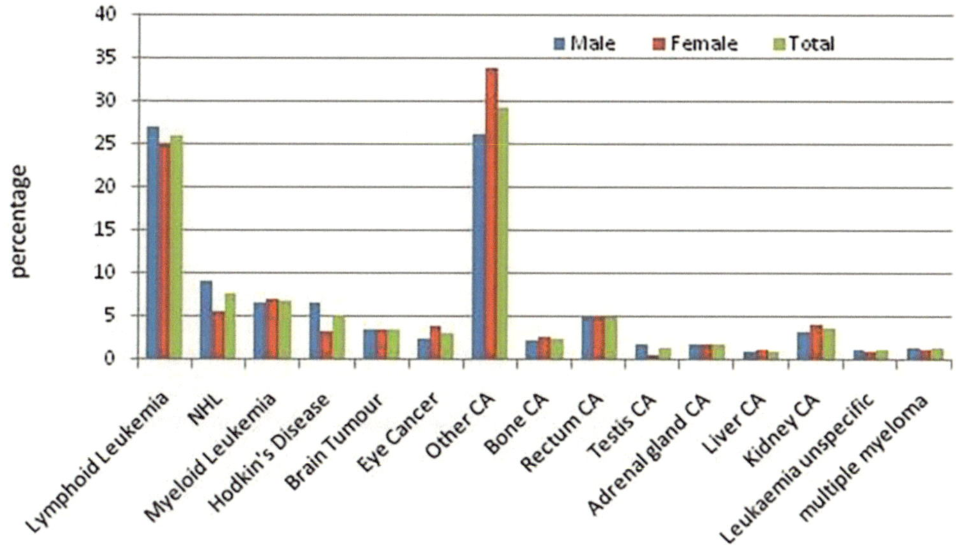

Figure 3.
Sex-wise distributions of reported cases and types of cancer (share in %).

Type of CA	00–04 Years	05–09 Years	10–14 Years
Lymphoid Leukemia	28.9	29.1	26.1
NHL	4.7	9.0	7.7
Myeloid Leukemia	14.7	3.7	6.8
Hodgkin's Disease	1.7	7.0	5.3
Brain Tumor	2.5	5.2	3.6
Eye Cancer	6.4	2.0	3.1
Other Cancer	24.3	27.5	29.3
Bone Cancer	.5	1.3	2.5
Rectum Cancer	3.9	5.1	5.0
Testis Cancer	.6	2.3	1.4
Adrenal gland Cancer	3.8	0.8	1.8
Liver Cancer	2.3	0.5	1.0
Kidney Cancer	3.1	4.2	3.7
Leukemia unspecific	1.0	1.3	1.2
Multiple myeloma	1.5	1.0	1.4
Total	100	100	100

Table 5.
Incidence of pediatric cancer across age group (share in %).

4. Conclusion

The analysis covers three thousand eight hundred and thirty-four cases of pediatric cancer registered at Madras Metropolitan Tumor Registry from 1982 to 2016.

Overall, the results indicate a gradual decline in childhood cancer during this period and indicate that maximum cases are reported during 2007–2011. The results confirm some of the established patterns including a higher incidence of cancer among male children (60.3%), and a high incidence among the children in 0–4 yearsage group. Leukemia is the most common pediatric cancer and it constitutes 27 percent in males and 25 percent in females. Overall cancers are more reported in the Hindu community, while specific types like myeloid leukemia, NHL, brain tumor, and multiple myeloma are found high in the Jain community. Lymphoid leukemia and rectum ca are more common in the Muslim community.

The pediatric tumor showed wide variation concerning different age groups. The genetic and environmental factors played role in the etiology of pediatric cancer. Most pediatric cancer is curable if it has been detected early. Thus, the study offers some important insights and updates on the pediatric cancer trends in the city of Chennai and may serve as a reference source for clinicians and researchers on pediatric oncology and policymakers engaged in public health.

Author details

Sajna Panolan*, Srinivas Govindarajulu, S. Kalpana, Valarmathi Srinivasan and Joseph Maria Adaikalam
The Tamil Nadu Dr. M.G.R. Medical University, Chennai, Tamil Nadu, India

*Address all correspondence to: sachusajnap@gmail.com

References

[1] Swaminathan R, Rama R, Shanta V. Childhood cancers in Chennai, India, 1990-2001: Incidence and survival. International journal of cancer. 2008;**122**(11):2607-2611

[2] Barr R, Riberio R, Agarwal B, Masera G, Hesseling P, Magrath I. Pediatric oncology in countries with limited resources. In: Pizzo PA, Poplack DG, editors. Principles and Practice of Pediatric Oncology, 5thed. Philadelphia: Lippincott Williams and Wilkins; 2006. pp. 1605-1617

[3] WHO. 10 facts about cancer. Available from: http://www.who.int/features/factfiles/cancer/03_en.html. [Accessed: March 10, 2019]

[4] Kramarova E, Stiller CA. International classification of childhood cancer (ICCC). In: Parkin DM, Kramarova E, Draper GJ, Masuyer E, Michaelis J, Neglia S, Qureshi S, Stiller CA, editors. International Incidence of Childhood Cancer. Vol. 144. Lyon: International Agency for Research on Cancer, IARC Scientific Publication; 1998. pp. 2, 15-19

[5] Parkin DM, Whelan SL, Ferlay J, Teppo L, Thomas DB. Cancer Incidence in Five Continents. Vol. 8. Lyon: International Agency for Research on Cancer, IARC Scientific Publication No. 155; 2002

[6] Howard SC, Pedrosa M, Lins M, Pedrosa A, Pui CH, Ribeiro RC, et al. Establishment of a pediatric oncology program and outcomes of childhood acute lymphoblastic leukemia in a resource-poor area. JAMA. 2004;**291**:2471-2475

[7] Harif M, Barsaoui S, Benchekroun S, Bouhas R, Doumbé P, Khattab M, et al. Treatment of B-cell lymphoma with LMB modified protocols in Africa--report of the French-African pediatric oncology group (GFAOP). Pediatric Blood & Cancer. 2008;**50**:1138-1142

[8] Arora RS, Eden TO, Kapoor G. Epidemiology of childhood cancer in India. Indian journal of cancer. 2009;**46**(4):264

[9] WHO. Health Situation in the South East Asia Region 1994-1997. New Delhi: Regional Office for SEAR; 1999

[10] Magrath I, Litvak J. Cancer in developing countries: Opportunity and challenge. Journal of the National Cancer Institute. 1993;**85**(11):862-874

[11] WHO. World Health Report 1999, Making a Difference. Report of the Director General. Geneva: WHO; 1999

[12] Mohan S, Asthana S, Labani S, Popli G. Cancer trends in India: A review of population-based cancer registries (2005-2014). Indian Journal of Public Health. 2018;**62**(3):221

[13] Srinath Reddy K, Shah B, Varghese C, Ramadoss A. Responding to the threat of chronic diseases in India. Lancet. 2005;**366**:1744-1749

[14] India. Office of the Registrar General, University of Toronto. Centre for Global Health Research. Report on Causes of Death in India, 2001-2003. Office of the Registrar General India in collaboration with Centre for Global Health Research, St. Michael's Hospital, University of Toronto; 2009.

[15] Bhutani M, Vora A, Kumar L, Kochupillai V. Lympho-hemopoietic malignancies in India. Medical Oncology. 2002;**19**(3):141-150

[16] Parkin DM. International variation. Oncogene. 2004;**23**(38):6329

[17] Das S, Paul DK, Anshu K, Bhakta S. Childhood cancer incidence in India between 2012 and 2014: Report of a population-based cancer registry. Indian Pediatrics. 2017;**54**(12):1033-1036

[18] Stiller C, editor. Childhood Cancer in Britain: Incidence Survival, Mortality. Oxford: Oxford University Press; 2007

[19] Gurney JG, Bondy ML. Epidemiology of childhood cancer. In: Pizzo PA, Poplack DG, editors. Priciples and Practice of Pediatric Oncology. 5th ed. Philadelphia: Lippincott Williams and Wilkins; 2006. pp. 2-14

Section 2

Role of Immune Cells and Metabolism in Cancer

Chapter 4

Perspective Chapter: Dendritic Cells in the Tumor Microenvironment

Dan Jin, Laura Falceto Font and Catherine T. Flores

Abstract

Tumor infiltrating dendritic cells (DCs) play a critical role in initiating the process of anti-tumor immune responses. They can uptake tumor antigens either directly at the tumor site or from circulating antigens, and elicit T cell activation and adaptive immunity in secondary lymphoid organs. Subtypes of dendritic cells have various roles in immunity and tumor rejection. In this chapter, we will summarize the role of dendritic cell populations on mounting anti-tumor immunity. Conversely, we will discuss tumor-mediated dysfunction of dendritic cells that aid immune evasion including prevention of recruitment, impairment in antigen presenting and mediation of tolerance. At last, we briefly introduced the progress in DC vaccine applications in clinic.

Keywords: dendritic cell, tumor microenvironment, antigen presenting, T cell activation, DC tolerance, DC vaccine

1. Introduction

Dendritic cells (DC) are responsible for activating effector responses and mediating adaptive immunity. Immune responses are dependent on multiple factors including the DC type, maturation status, and immunogenicity of antigens. DCs have the capacity of inducing protective immunity as well as generating a tolerogenic immune environment. The complexity of how cancer impacts the spectrum of response varies depending on the cancer type, largely on the cancer immunophenotype. Here we discuss how different DC subtypes interact between cancer and adaptive immunity. We also touch on various cancer-mediated immune evasion strategies that alter DC function. Lastly we evaluate immunotherapeutic strategies that employ DCs to elicit anti-tumor T cell responses.

2. Anti-tumor roles of different dendritic cell sub-populations

DCs are composed of heterogenous sub-populations with each subtype possessing unique functions to compensate for each other. They cooperate to elicit both innate and adaptive immunity. In this section, we will generally review the roles of different DC sub-populations in anti-tumor immunity (**Figure 1**).

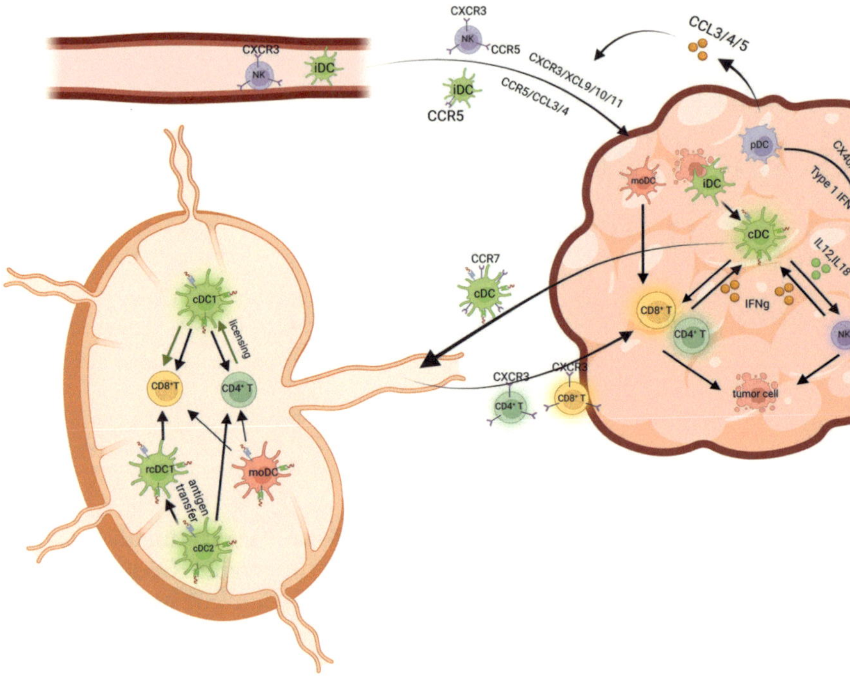

Figure 1.
Roles of DC subpopulations in anti-tumor response. Immature DCs in peripheral tissue can be recruited into tumor site through CCR5/CCL3/4 chemoaxis. Both cDC1 and cDC2 uptake tumor antigens in situ and migrate to tdLN in a CCR7-dependent way, trafficking tumor antigens into tdLN. In tdLN, antigen-loaded cDC1 primes both naïve CD8 T cells and CD4 T cells. Primed CD4 T cells further boost CD8 T cell activation through licensing cDC1 in a CD40/CD40L dependent way. Antigen-loaded cDC2 predominantly primes naïve CD4 T cells. It can alternatively activate CD8 T cells through transferring antigens to LN resident cDC1(rcDC1), which primes naïve T cells in LN. Activated T cells migrate to tumor site in a CXCR3 dependent chemokine recruitment way. Effector T cells can be further stimulated by antigen activated cDCs and moDCs in tumor and exert cytotoxic tumor killing. moDCs exert CD4 and CD8 T priming function to compensate for cDCs when they are dysfunctional or depleted. Activated pDCs secrete CCL chemokines to recruit and activate NK cells through type I IFN and OX40-OX40L interaction. Activated NK cells promote cytotoxic CD8 T priming through activation of cDC in an IFNγ-dependent way, meanwhile, activated cDCs secrete cytokines like IL12, IL18 that enhance NK cell activation.

2.1 Conventional DCs

Conventional DCs (cDCs) are derived from common DC precursors (CDP) in the bone marrow, which are comprised of two main subsets: cDC1 and cDC2. The infiltration of cDCs in the tumor has a positive correlation with patient survival in some solid cancers [1]. cDC1 development is specified by transcriptional factors BATF3, IRF8, and ID2, while cDC2 development depends on transcriptional factors RELB, IRF4, ZEB2 and KLF4 [2, 3]. BATF3 is required for maintaining IRF8 expression during cDC1 commitment in specified cDC1 progenitor [4]. BATF3 is also required for cDC1 cross-presentation function and cross-presentation independent anti-tumor immunity functions [5, 6]. BATF-dependent cDC1 is specified by its unique role to initiate naïve $CD8^+$ T cell activation in tumor-draining lymph nodes(tdLN), as well as enhance both T cell accumulation and local CD8 T cell cytotoxicity. The abundance of cDC1 in the tumor microenvironment positively correlates with cancer patient survival and response to immunotherapy across different cancer types [7, 8]. $CD103^+$ cDC1s sample tumor antigen in tumor mass and migrate to tumor-draining lymph nodes via CCR7, where they prime T cell responses [9]. Tumor-resident $BATF3^+$ cDC1s secret CXCL9 and CXCL10 to recruit CXCR3 expressing effector T cells and NK cells [10, 11]. In turn, IFNγ produced by tumor effector T cells and NK cells induce CXCL9/10/11 production by myeloid cells, creating a feedback loop in this response [12]. cDCs also secrete IL-12, IL-18 and IL-2 provoking NK cells to produce IFNγ, TNFα, or GM-CSF, which further promotes DC activation [13].

Unlike cDC1s, cDC2s have limited capacity to cross-present tumor antigens to CD8 T cells. The function of cDC2s are largely restricted to priming of CD4 T cells in tdLN or in tumor [14–16]. cDC2s mediate cross-presentation of soluble antigens and is enhanced by TLR7 agonist [17, 18]. cDC2s complement the function of cDC1s by also activating CD8 T cells. Migratory cDC2 capture antigens in tumor and transfer antigens to LN resident cDC1s through antigen vesicles and synaptic transfer, which is capable of activating CD8 T cells [19]. In the absence of cDC1s, activating cDC2s by type I IFN can stimulate CD8 T activation in tumor [20]. In preclinical models where cDC1 function is impaired, deletion of cDC1 population improves cDC2 migration into tdLN and CD4 T activation [1].

2.2 Plasmacytoid dendritic cells

Plasmacytoid dendritic cells(pDC) are largely regarded as immunomodulating cells through secretion of massive amounts of type-I interferon during anti-virus immune responses. The role of pDC in anti-tumor immunity is controversial. pDC in tumors have been found to have impaired response to Toll-like receptor activation and decreased type-I IFN production. They recruit and expand immune regulatory T cells in the tumor microenvironment (TME) and are associated with poor prognosis [15, 21]. As an escape mechanism, tumor cells attract pDCs to induce an immunosuppressive environment through secreting chemokine CXCL12 [22].

On the contrary, in some solid tumors, pharmacological agents can be used to overcome immunosuppression. For example, imiquimod stimulation can induce pDC mediated tumor killing via secretion of TRAIL and granzyme B independent of adaptive immunity [23]. pDCs can also drive anti-tumor response by activating adaptive T cell immunity mediated by cDC activation dependent on type-I IFN [24]. Direct injection of TLR9 activated pDC into B16 melanoma tumor bearing mice induces robust cytotoxic T lymphocytes (CTL) cross priming against tumor, leading to tumor regression. TLR9 activated pDCs produce large amounts of chemokines CCL3, CCL4, and CCL5 within the tumor, which recruits $CCR5^+$ NK cells. Recruited NK cells are activated by pDC through cell-to-cell interaction via OX40/OX40L and type I IFN secreted by pDC. Tumor cells lysated by NK cells cause tumor antigen release into cDCs and IFNg secreted by activated NK cells also help activate CTL in dLN [25]. Such an activated subset of pDC with higher levels of OX40 is also found in head and neck squamous cell carcinoma (HNSCC) tumor with distinct immunostimulatory and cytolytic function and can synergize with cDCs in generating tumor antigen-specific $CD8^+$ T cell responses [26].

2.3 Monocyte-derived dendritic cells

Monocyte-derived dendritic cells (moDCs) are differentiated from monocytes under inflammatory conditions. Activation of p53 in MDSCs and monocytic progenitors can induce moDC-like population differentiation in tumor, which potentiates the anti-tumor response [27]. Increase of moDC in tdLN can be a measurable indication of immune activation, particularly after treatment with pharmacological agents such as TLR agonists [28]. moDCs in tumor are essential for CD8 T activation and antitumor response after local immunostimulatory agent treatment [29]. In mice with Zbtb46-DTR bone marrow chimeras, which are deficient in cDC production after diphtheria toxin (DT) treatment, moDC compensate for the loss of cDCs and account for intratumoral CTL expansion and function [30]. Compared with cDC, moDCs are less efficient at inducing CD4 T cell proliferation but more efficient at inducing Th1 and Th17 differentiation [31]. However, moDCs are also able to cross-present antigens through the vacuolar pathway and activate naïve CD4 T and CD8 T cells [32]. *In vitro* differentiated moDCs have been used in clinical trials as vaccines for cancer patients and encouraging responses have been shown when combined with other cancer therapies [33–37], which will be further discussed in the last section of this chapter.

3. Tumor-mediated immune evasion: impact on dendritic cells

3.1 DC tumor infiltration and migration to LN

cDCs in tumor are found to be sparse among tumor infiltrated immune populations [8, 38]. Increased cDC amount within tumor is associated with improved prognosis and response to check-point inhibitor immunotherapy [8, 39]. Tumor cells secret soluble factors that suppress DCs infiltrating to tumor site and migrating to LN (**Figure 2**).

Tumor cells suppress chemokine CCL4 production through activating beta-catenin signaling, and beta-catenin activation induces ATF3 expression. ATF3 binds the promoter of CCL4 gene and suppresses CCL4 expression. Decreased CCL4 leads to decreased intratumoral cDC recruitment by CCL4/CCR5 axis [40]. beta-catenin signaling suppresses CCL5 level in tumor loci. CCL5/CCR5 chemoaxis recruits cDC1 into tumor. Increased CCL5 expression in tumor recruits cDC tumoral infiltration and promotes anti-tumor immune response and promotes efficacy when combined with anti-PD1 [41]. Prostaglandin E2 (PGE2), a prostanoid lipid catalyzed by enzyme cyclooxygenase (COX), is highly produced in tumor [42–44]. cDC1s are absent from

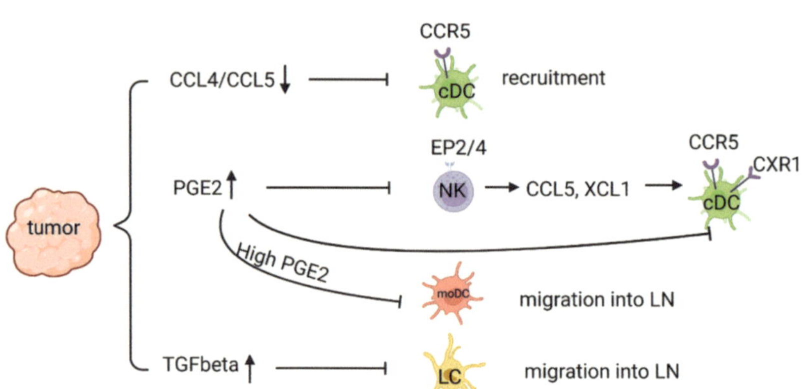

Figure 2.
Impact of DC recruitment and migration by tumor. Tumor cells suppress CCL4/5 expression by inducing β-catenin signaling pathway, which inhibits cDC recruitment via CCL4/5/CCR5 chemoaxis. PGE2 produced from tumor directly acts on intratumoral NK cells through EP2/4 receptors. PGE2 inhibits CCL5 and XCL1 secretion by NK cells, which results in decreased cDC recruitment. PGE2 can also inhibit CCR5 and CXR1 expression on cDC to impair cDC recruitment. High concentration of PGE2 inhibits moDC migration into dLN. TGFβ from tumor inhibits LC migration into LN.

PGE2 producing tumor. PGE2 suppresses NK cells mediated cDC1 recruitment in tumor. Intratumoral NK cells secret cDC1 chemoattractant CCL5, XCL1, which are inhibited by tumor derived PGE2 through PGE2 receptor EP2, EP4 on NK cells. However, expressing CCL5, or XCL1 in tumor is insufficient to reverse intratumoral DC exclusion in PGE2 producing tumor. Further study shows that PGE2 can also downregulate CXR1 and CCR5 expression in DC, which leads to impairment of response to chemokine even in the existence of chemoattractant [21, 44, 45].

DC cells uptake antigens in tumor site and then migrate to dLN for priming T cells. TGFβ secreted from tumor inhibits DC migration to dLN in both autocrine and paracrine way. Langerhans cells (LCs), skin-resident DCs, play critical role in eliciting immune response in skin disease. Besides of tumor cells, LCs are also active TGFβ producer. Knock-out of TGFβ or its receptor in LCs induces mass migration of LCs to regional LN in both steady and inflammation states [46]. In skin tumor model, TGFβ inhibits tumor infiltration and migration to skin-dLN by LCs [47]. Role of PGE2 in regulating DC migration relies on its concentration. High concentration of PGE2 suppresses DC migration while it has also been shown as a positive regulator of CCR7 expression and migration of moDCs [48, 49].

3.2 Antigen presentation

Tumor cells develop mechanisms to impair antigen capture and presenting by DCs (**Figure 3**). Molecules released or exposed from dying cancer cells can act as danger signals to circulating DCs. DCs recognize dying/dead tumor cells or tumor derived debris through danger-associated molecular patterns (DAMPs) mediated by pattern recognition receptors (PRRs) like TLRs, and phagocyze dying-tumor cells or tumor derived debris [50]. DAMPs include ATP, heat shock proteins (HSPs), HMGB1, calreticulin, annexin A1, dsDNA, but are not limited to these [50]. Antigen uptake will stimulate DC maturation and migration to dLN. Internalized antigens will be processed and presented on the DC surface by MHC-I and MHC-II molecules. MHC-I molecules used to be thought for intracellular peptide presenting, while MHC-II is for exogenous peptide. However, this is not always the case. Cross-presenting is termed for presenting exogenous antigens by MHC-I, which plays a critical role in eliciting anti-tumor immune response by DCs [51]. Proteins internalized by DCs are degraded in phagosomes into peptides [52]. Peptides are then translocated into endoplasmic reticulum (ER) by transporter associated with antigen presentation (TAP). The MHC-I heterodimer is assembled in ER from a polymorphic heavy chain and a light chain β2-microglobulin (β2m) and stabilized by chaperone proteins like calreticulin and tapasin when peptide is not loaded. Chaperones will be exchanged when peptide is loaded. Peptides fit into the MHC-I peptide binding groove which stabilizes the peptide-MHC-I complex. MHC-II comprises transmembrane α- and β-chains and an invariant chain. MHC-II will be transported to a MHC-II compartment, an endosomal compartment, for invariant chain digestion, resulting a class II-associated lipid peptide (CLIP). With the help of H2-DM/HLA-DM, CLIP is exchanged with antigen peptide [53]. In LN, DCs present tumor antigens to CD8 T cells and CD4 T cells dependent on MHC-I and MHC-II respectively. Tumor proteins will be processed into immunogenic peptides and loaded on MHC-I or MHC-II molecules on cell surface.

Tumor cells evolved multiple immune escape strategies to prevent recognition by DCs. For example, tumor-derived stanniocalcin 1(STC1) interacts with DAMP signal, calreticulin (CRT), to prevent CRT membrane from exposing to APCs, thereby abrogating membrane CRT-directed phagocytosis by DCs. High expression of STC1

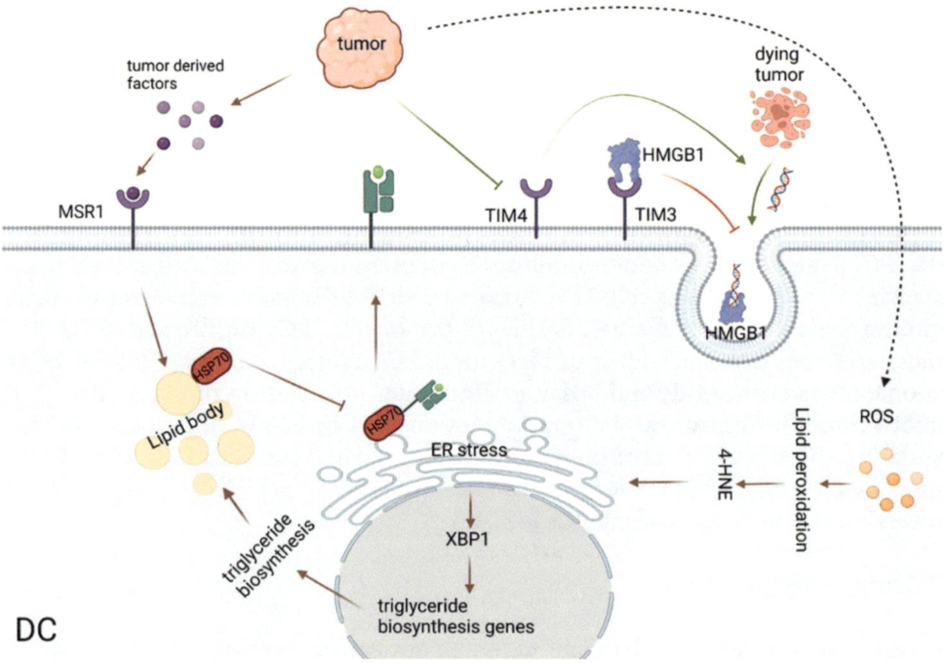

Figure 3.
Tumor induced impairment of DC on tumor antigen capture and presentation. Tumor derived factors mediate lipid body accumulation in DC by inducing MSR1 expression. ROS, induced by tumor microenvironment, leads to increase lipid peroxidation in DC. Byproduct of lipid peroxidation, 4-HNE, induces ER stress, which activates XBP1 transcription factor. XBP1 then increases genes synthesizing triglyceride. Increased triglyceride leads to increased oxidized lipid bodies. The lipid bodies competitively bind HSP70 with pMHC, preventing pMHC been translocated onto cell surface. TIM3 competitively binds HMGB1 with dying tumor derive DNA, inhibiting DNA stimulated immune response via preventing DNA been internalized into DC. Tumor inhibits TIM4 expression on DC, thus inhibiting TIM4 mediated tumor associated antigen capture.

in tumor is significantly correlated with poor responses to immunotherapy in patients [54]. In another immune escape mechanism, the mevalonate (MVA) pathway, which is highly activated in tumor cells, reduces F-actin exposure, a DAMP signal, on tumor cells, evading recognition mediated by Clec9A on cDC1. The MVA increases protein geranylgeranylation on Rac1, a small GTPase controlling actin cytoskeleton, resulting reduced F-actin in tumor [55–57]. The immune modulator TIM-3 is also highly expressed by DCs and has been shown to play an inhibitory role on DC activation. TIM-3 inhibits tumor derived DNA uptake by cDC1 through inhibiting endocytosis. HMGB1, a ligand of TIM-3, also acts as a DAMPS signal and binds tumor-derived DNA and is taken up by DCs. TIM-3 inhibits this process through sequestering HMGB1 bound DNA on cell surface [58]. TIM4, another T- cell immunoglobulin and mucin domain gene as TIM3, is also expressed on APCs like macrophages and dendritic cells. DAMP signal induces TIM4 expression on intratumoral macrophages and DCs [59]. Though TIM4 on tumor associated macrophage (TAM) has been shown impedes tumor antigen presentation through activating autophagy in TAM upon tumor antigen uptake in mouse melanoma model [59], TIM4 on lung resident cDCs in lung adenocarcinoma model shows a positive role in promoting anti-tumor immune activation [60]. TIM4 expression is downregulated in cDC1 from advanced lung tumor. Blocking TIM4 or knocking out of TIM4 abolishes tumor antigen uptake by lung resident cDC1 and impairs antigen presenting to CD8 T cells in vitro and in vivo.

DCs from tumor-bearing host have been found with accumulated lipids. Tumor derived factors induce oxidized lipid accumulation in cDCs from tumor bearing host. DCs have high oxidized lipids shows impaired cross-presentation while not affecting presenting endogenous antigens, and nor affecting the level of MHC-I. Scavenger receptor, MSR1, induced by tumor derived factors, accounts for the lipid accumulation in DC [61, 62]. ER stress signaling also involved in oxidized lipid accumulation in DC from tumor bearing host. 4-HNE is a byproduct from lipid peroxidation mediated by ROS and triggers ER stress and XBP1 activation. XBP1, a multitask transcription factor in response to ER stress, induces triglyceride biosynthesis. Elevated triglyceride biosynthesis leads to accumulated abnormal lipids and suppresses DC function [63]. HSP70 is a chaperon protein that binds with pMHC, and facilitates pMHC trafficking onto cell surface. Oxidative lipid bodies, not non-oxidized lipid bodies, competitively bind HSP70 covalently, preclude HSP70 interaction with pMHC, thus affect pMHC trafficking to cell surface [64].

3.3 Tolerance

Tumor cells have evolved different mechanisms to promote DC tolerance to facilitate immune escape (**Figure 4**). Tolerized DCs experience higher co-inhibitory markers, including PD-L1, PD-L2 and higher arginase activity, and lower MHC-II and co-stimulation markers, including CD80, CD86, CD40 [39, 65]. Tolerized DCs are not capable of activating T cells, while promote immune suppression through mechanisms like, for example, Treg upregulation.

3.3.1 Secreted factors from tumor environment

Secreted tumor-derived factors is one of the major ways of driving DC tolerance, these include PGE2 and TGFβ which lead to subsequent induction of other immune modifiers. Tumor derived PGE2 suppresses cDCs activation by suppressing co-stimulation, IL-12 production, and increasing PD-L1 and Arg1 [44, 66]. PGE2 is the main inducer of arginase-1 during tumor induced DC tolerization [67]. TGFβ from

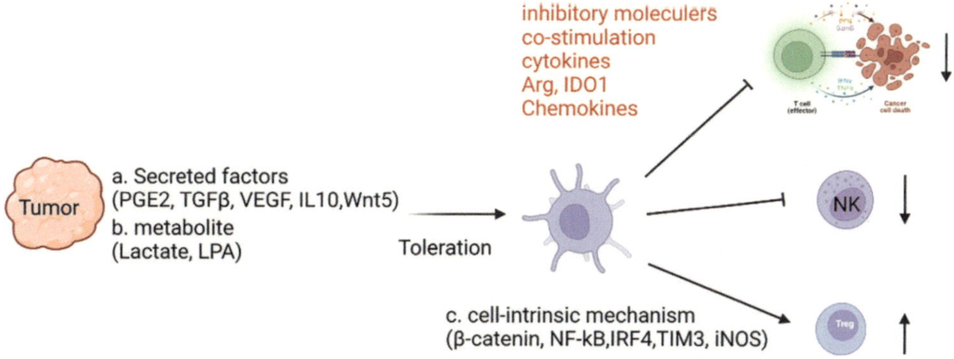

Figure 4.
DC tolerance mechanism. Secreted factors or metabolites derived from tumor environment induce dendritic cell tolerance through activating or inhibiting cell-intrinsic signaling pathways in DC. DC tolerance leads to induced inhibitory molecular expression, Arg and IDO1 upregulation, anti-inflammation cytokine production and suppress co-stimulation and pro-inflammation cytokine production. And also result into dysregulated chemokine secretion. DC tolerance abolishes anti-tumor immune response through inhibiting T cell and NK recruitment and mediated tumor killing, and promoting immunosuppressive Treg differentiation and recruitment.

tumor also induces DC tolerization [67, 68]. TGFβ induces IDO expression in pDC and enhances expression of CCL22 by myeloid DCs in tumor. IDO suppresses effector T cell activity and promotes Treg differentiation and activation. DC-derived CCL22 chemokine promotes CCR4-dependent recruitment of Tregs to the tumor microenvironment [69]. pDCs in tumor environments are associated with poor survival. Co-culture with TGFβ containing medium inhibits pDC activation and type I IFN secretion. Tolerized pDCs promote tumor growth through inhibiting NK cell infiltration and recruitment of Treg cells [70]. DCs with high TGFβ expression are poor at eliciting the activation of naive CD4 T cells and sustaining their proliferation and differentiation into Th1 effectors. Vascular endothelial growth factor (VEGF) inhibits LPS induced DC maturation via Nrp-1 receptor on DC. NRP1 interacted with LPS receptor TLR4 and suppressed downstream ERK and NF-κβ signaling, resulting in increased expression of MHC-II and costimulatory molecules (CD40, CD86) as well as proinflammatory cytokine production inhibition [71]. Infiltrating macrophages were the primary source of IL-10 within tumors, blocking IL-10 signaling increases intratumoral dendritic cell expression of IL-12 during chemotherapy in breast cancer [65].

LPA is a bioactive lipid produced by tumor cells. Blocking LPA-generating enzyme autotaxin in ovarian cancer cells elicits anti-tumor immune response driven by type-I IFN. LPA induces PGE2 synthesis by DCs, which suppressed type-I IFN production and response in DC via autocrine EP4 engagement [72]. Lactate is an oncometabolite resulted from metabolic adaption in cancer cells via Warburg effect. Lactate in tumor attenuates pDC activation in response to TLR9 ligand and consequent type I IFN induction. pDC tolerization by lactate is partially through activating GPR81, a cell surface G-protein coupled receptor of lactate. GPR81 activation induces intracellular $Ca2^{+}$ mobilization and activates calcineurin phosphatase (CALN) expression. Inhibition of CALN reverses the inhibitory effect by lactate. Extracellular lactate can also influence pDCs through intracellular import via the monocarboxylate transporters (MCT). Inhibition of MCT genes resulte in significant reversal of the lactate-mediated inhibition of IFNα. Thus, both GPR81 triggering and cytosolic import via the MCT transporters mechanism are involved in lactate induced pDC tolerization. Lactate treated pDCs have enhanced tryptonphan metabolism, leading to excessive production of kynurenines which in turn induces Treg cell differentiation [73].

3.3.2 Cell-intrinsic mechanism

Tumor-derived Wnt5a induces β-catenin signaling activation-dependent IDO expression in DCs. DCs conditioned by wnt5a promote Treg development and suppresses effector T cell activation [74, 75]. β-Catenin complexed with PPAR-γ upon wnt5a stimulation and transcriptionally activates fatty acid oxidation (FAO) synthesis gene, CPT1a, inducing the synthesis of heme prosthetic group, protoporphyrin IX, which is required for IDO enzymatic activity [75]. Wnt1/β-catenin signaling in DC suppresses chemokine production, leading to T cell exclusion in tumor and decreased T cell activation [76]. β-catenin signaling in DC also impairs CD8 T priming through inducing IL-10 secretion via mTOR activation. Even though the negative regulation of initial CD8 T priming by β-catenin/mTOR/IL10 in DC, β-catenin–regulated IL-10 also shown has an opposite anti-tumor immunity role through maintenance of primed CD8 T cells after clonal expansion [77, 78]. β-catenin can also interact with TCF4 and activates gene expression of Aldh1, an enzyme to produce retinoic acid (RA) from vitamin A, resulting increased RA in DC [79]. Aldh1 expression in mature DC significantly correlated with immunoregulatory module including genes like PD-L1, PD-L2, CD83, and CCL22 [80]. RA induces Treg generation in vitro and in vivo [81–83]. DC maturation suppression could be mediated by E-cadherin based DC-DC adhesion. Disrupting this contact activates DC maturation through activating β-catenin/TCF, leading to increase of co-stimulatory molecules, MHC-II and chemokine receptors. However, such DC maturation is not coupled with proinflammation cytokine secretion and failed to prime CD4 T cells, coupled with a distinct transcriptional profile from those induced by TLR activation. DC matured by E-cadherin disruption also leads to Treg production. The data suggests a DC function regulatory role of E-cadherin/β-catenin/TCF axis [84].

Nuclear factor-κB (NF-κB) is an important transcription factor that participating in cancer inflammation. There are two general types of NF-κB signaling pathways: canonical and non-canonical pathways [85]. Canonical and non-canonical NF-κB pathways play different roles in DC functional regulation. Lung cancer patient derived tumor sera induce canonical NF-κB pathway inhibition, while activates non-canonical NF-kB pathway in human mo-DC [86]. IFNγ has been shown important for myeloid activation [87]. Canonical NF-κb/IRF1 mediated IFNγ response pathway is required for intra-tumoral cDC1 activation. IFNγ knock out or IFNGR1 knock out in cDC1 abolished IL12 production [88]. Impaired NF-κB or IRF1 loses control of tumor growth and expression of maturation markers and chemokines (CXCL9/10) for recruiting T cells [89]. Inhibiting NF-κB in BMDC has no effect on MHC-II or co-stimulation molecules, while promotes Treg differentiation in vitro [80]. VEGF mediated inhibition on LPS stimulated BMDC activation is dependent on the inhibition of canonical NF-κB signaling pathway [66]. Noncanonical NF-kB signaling in dendritic cells is required for IDO induction in the late stage of DC activation by CD40 ligation [90].

Inhibitory molecular expression on DC suppresses T cell activation and induces Treg differentiation. PD-L1 upregulation in tolerized DC is not dependent on the presence of type I and type II IFN signaling, nor is dependent on inflammasome or TRIF/MyD88 signaling. Instead, PD-L1 upregulation is dependent on phagocytic cell-surface receptor AXL activation upon antigen uptake. IL-4 signaling negatively regulates IL-12 production on DC. Blocking IL-4 signaling can increase IL-12 production without upregulating PD-L1 [88]. IRF4 plays a dural role of upregulating antigen presenting capability and tolerization of BMDC. Depletion of IRF4 reduces Aldh1 and PD-L2 expression, coupled with elevated cytokine IL-12 an TNF expression. IRF4-deficient DC is impaired for Treg generation in vivo. TIM-3 is predominantly found expressed in cDC cells in tumor. TIM-3 expression on DC can be induced by IL-10 or VEGF [91]. Blocking TIM-3 improve survival when combined with chemotherapy. The regulatory effect by TIM-3 blocking is neither through affecting cDC infiltration nor through regulating cDC activation. However, TIM-3 blocking increases CXCL9 secretion by cDC1, which is a ligand for CXCR3. CXCL9/CXCR3 chemoaxis attracts T cells into tumor [92]. TIM-3 on DC impaires DC recognition and response to tumor derived nucleic acids. TIM-3 serves as a receptor for DNA sensor, HMGB1, completing with nucleic acids for binding to th A-box domain of HMGB1. The binding of TIM-3 on HMGB1 inhibits nucleic acids to be internalized into endosomes [87].

DC activation is accompanied by an increased glycolysis metabolic process, which is required by both survival and effector function of activated DC. Bioactive gas nitric oxide (NO) is synthesized and secreted by activated DC, playing an immunomodulating role of DC. Cellular production of NO is catalyzed by NOS enzymes, which converts substrates L-arginine, NADPH and O2 to L-citrulline, NADP+, and NO [93]. Inducible NOS (iNOS) is the primary NO-synthesizing enzyme expressed by DC. iNOS expression in $CD103^{-}CD11b^{+}$ intratumoral DC is required for tumor suppressive Th17 T cell differentiation in PDA model [94]. Glucose could inhibit DC function through mTOR/HIF1a/iNOS signaling axis, inhibiting co-stimulation molecular expression and IL12 secretion and restricting T cell activation. When T cells encounter DCs, they compete for glucose availability, which suppress the glucose sensitive pathway resulting T cell activation [95]. Monocyte-derived tumor associated DCs are prominent in tumor antigen uptake, but lack of strong T-cell stimulatory capacity due to NO-mediated immunosuppression [96].

4. Application of DC vaccine in tumor immunotherapy

4.1 DC vaccination

DCs are the most efficient professional antigen-presenting cells that can initiate an adaptive immune response by presenting antigens to T cells [97, 98]. In the past 25 years, many groups have exploited this characteristic to create dendritic cell vaccines to direct the immune system to fight cancer. DC cell-based vaccine approaches have been proved safe for their minimal toxicity, and their low association rates with autoimmunity [99, 100]. The general process of DC vaccine preparation including DC generation, antigen loading and DC maturation. To date, different strategies have been developed to generate DC vaccine for clinical applications.

The most commonly used approach to generate DCs is through ex-vivo differentiation from peripheral blood. The advantage of this method is the easy generation of sufficient autologous DCs for vaccination. However, therapeutic outcomes still have a lot of room for improvement, with less than 15% the patients showing objective response [101]. Due to the artificial *in vitro* differentiation process, moDCs have compromised functionality compared with naturally-occurring DCs with different transcriptional profiles. The limitation of using naturally-occurring DCs is the low frequency of DCs in peripheral blood, resulting in a highly labor-intensive process in DC isolation for clinical use. To overcome this, a growing effort in the field has been exerted to facilitate the developing a feasible protocol, for example, an automatic system that can prepare DCs [102]. For DC vaccine production, DCs are then be loaded with total tumor lysate or RNAs and tumor associated antigens. The loading methods include pulsing by co-culturing, electroporation, viral transduction or DC-tumor fusion [103]. Maturation cocktails used in the clinic consist of TLR agonists and cytokines, often in combination with co-stimulatory proteins like CD40L. Introducing mRNAs coding constitutively-active TLR4, CD40L and CD70 via electroporation has shown clinical success [33, 104].

4.2 DC vaccination clinical trial in glioblastoma

DC vaccination in the context of glioblastoma has shown both positive and negative results in clinical trials. Even though a phase III clinical trial aiming to assess DC vaccine targeting the EGFR deletion mutation EGFRvIII in newly diagnosed EGFRvIII-expressing GBM patients failed [105], some other clinical trials have shown promising results. Another phase III clinical trial utilizing an autologous tumor lysate-pulsed dendritic cell vaccine combined with standard therapy showed significant overall survival benefit from 15 to 17 months to 23.1 months [36]. In another phase II clinical trial, ICT-107 (autologous dendritic cells (DC) pulsed with six synthetic peptide epitopes targeting GBM tumor/stem cell-associated antigens MAGE-1, HER-2, AIM-2, TRP-2, gp100, and IL13Rα2 was given to newly diagnosed glioblastoma patients in addition to standard therapy. Results showed progression free survival (PFS) increased 2.2 months in ICT-107 cohort compared with matched DC control cohort. HLA-A2 subgroup patients achieved a meaningful therapeutic benefit with ICT-107, in both the MGMT methylated and unmethylated prespecified subgroups, whereas only HLA-A1 methylated patients had an OS benefit [106, 107]. Combination with other intervention methods could help increase DC vaccine efficacy. Pre-conditioning at vaccinated site can improve DC vaccination efficacy. Mitchell et al. (2015) showed that glioblastoma patients pre-exposed to tetanus/diphtheria (Td) toxoid in the vaccine site before vaccination with pp65 RNA-pulsed DCs had improved tumor-antigen-specific DC migration and improved survival compared to the ones that were not pre-exposed to the toxoid through increasing DC migration to dLN [108]. Three phase II clinical trials (ATTAC; ELEVATE; NCT00639639, NCT00639639, NCT02366728) aim to test pp65 DC with Td vaccine in newly diagnosed GBM patients. Results to date have shown that despite a small cohort, three successive trials demonstrate consistent survival outcomes, supporting the efficacy of *cytomegalovirus* DC vaccine therapy in GBM [109].

5. Conclusions

Dendritic cells, as the most professional APCs, play key roles in mediating the bridge between innate and adaptive immunity in anti-tumor immunity. DC subpopulations, through use of different action mechanisms in activating adaptive immunity, collaborate with each other to elicit anti-tumor immunity. In the battle with tumor, DC functions become regulated by tumor cells or other components in the tumor microenvironment, leading to DC dysfunction. These include impairments on antigen uptake, antigen presentation, migration to LN, and DC tolerance. Secreted factors from the tumor environment play a key role in mediating DC regulation. These suppressive signals act on DCs inducing DC dysfunction through different cellular intrinsic pathways. DC vaccine development for tumor treatment has made significant progress in the last decades, but still faces challenges in achieving a wide and significant therapeutic success. Deepening our understanding on DC function and regulation in the tumor environment will help the field in developing new and more powerful therapeutic intervention approaches.

Acknowledgements

This work was funded by NIH NINDS 5R01NS111033-03.

Conflict of interest

CF is a founder of iOncologi.

Author details

Dan Jin, Laura Falceto Font and Catherine T. Flores*
University of Florida, Gainesville, United States

*Address all correspondence to: catherine.flores@ufl.neurosurgery.edu

References

[1] Iwanowycz S et al. Type 2 dendritic cells mediate control of cytotoxic T cell resistant tumors. JCI Insight. 2021;**6**(17):e145885

[2] Amon L et al. Transcriptional control of dendritic cell development and functions. International Review of Cell and Molecular Biology. 2019;**349**:55-151

[3] Tussiwand R et al. Klf4 expression in conventional dendritic cells is required for T helper 2 cell responses. Immunity. 2015;**42**(5):916-928

[4] Grajales-Reyes GE et al. Batf3 maintains autoactivation of Irf8 for commitment of a CD8alpha(+) conventional DC clonogenic progenitor. Nature Immunology. 2015;**16**(7):708-717

[5] Hildner K et al. Batf3 deficiency reveals a critical role for CD8alpha+ dendritic cells in cytotoxic T cell immunity. Science. 2008;**322**(5904):1097-1100

[6] Theisen DJ et al. Batf3-dependent genes control tumor rejection induced by dendritic cells independently of cross-presentation. Cancer Immunology Research. 2019;**7**(1):29-39

[7] Bottcher JP, e Sousa CR. The role of Type 1 conventional dendritic cells in cancer immunity. Trends Cancer. 2018;**4**(11):784-792

[8] Broz ML et al. Dissecting the tumor myeloid compartment reveals rare activating antigen-presenting cells critical for T cell immunity. Cancer Cell. 2014;**26**(5):638-652

[9] Roberts EW et al. Critical role for CD103(+)/CD141(+) dendritic cells bearing CCR7 for tumor antigen trafficking and priming of t cell immunity in melanoma. Cancer Cell. 2016;**30**(2):324-336

[10] Spranger S et al. Tumor-residing Batf3 dendritic cells are required for effector T cell trafficking and adoptive T cell therapy. Cancer Cell. 2017;**31**(5):711-723 e4

[11] Wendel M et al. Natural killer cell accumulation in tumors is dependent on IFN-gamma and CXCR3 ligands. Cancer Research. 2008;**68**(20):8437-8445

[12] Metzemaekers M et al. Overview of the mechanisms that may contribute to the non-redundant activities of interferon-inducible CXC chemokine receptor 3 ligands. Frontiers in Immunology. 2017;**8**:1970

[13] Bodder J et al. Harnessing the cDC1-NK cross-talk in the tumor microenvironment to battle cancer. Frontiers in Immunology. 2020;**11**:631713

[14] Binnewies M et al. Unleashing Type-2 dendritic cells to drive protective antitumor CD4(+) T cell immunity. Cell. 2019;**177**(3):556-571 e16

[15] Verneau J, Sautes-Fridman C, Sun CM. Dendritic cells in the tumor microenvironment: Prognostic and theranostic impact. Seminars in Immunology. 2020;**48**:101410

[16] Ivashkiv LB. IFNgamma: Signalling, epigenetics and roles in immunity, metabolism, disease and cancer immunotherapy. Nature Reviews Immunology. 2018;**18**(9):545-558

[17] Theisen DJ et al. WDFY4 is required for cross-presentation in response to viral and tumor antigens. Science. 2018;**362**(6415):694-699

[18] Desch AN et al. Dendritic cell subsets require cis-activation for cytotoxic CD8 T-cell induction. Nature Communications. 2014;**5**:4674

[19] Ruhland MK et al. Visualizing synaptic transfer of tumor antigens among dendritic cells. Cancer Cell. 2020;**37**(6):786-799 e5

[20] Duong E et al. Type I interferon activates MHC class I-dressed CD11b(+) conventional dendritic cells to promote protective anti-tumor CD8(+) T cell immunity. Immunity. 2022;**55**(2): 308-323 e9

[21] Bottcher JP et al. NK cells stimulate recruitment of cDC1 into the tumor microenvironment promoting cancer immune control. Cell. 2018;**172**(5):1022-1037 e14

[22] Zou W et al. Stromal-derived factor-1 in human tumors recruits and alters the function of plasmacytoid precursor dendritic cells. Nature Medicine. 2001;**7**(12):1339-1346

[23] Drobits B et al. Imiquimod clears tumors in mice independent of adaptive immunity by converting pDCs into tumor-killing effector cells. The Journal of Clinical Investigation. 2012;**122**(2):575-585

[24] Nierkens S et al. Immune adjuvant efficacy of CpG oligonucleotide in cancer treatment is founded specifically upon TLR9 function in plasmacytoid dendritic cells. Cancer Research. 2011;**71**(20):6428-6437

[25] Liu C et al. Plasmacytoid dendritic cells induce NK cell-dependent, tumor antigen-specific T cell cross-priming and tumor regression in mice. The Journal of Clinical Investigation. 2008;**118**(3):1165-1175

[26] Poropatich K et al. OX40+ plasmacytoid dendritic cells in the tumor microenvironment promote antitumor immunity. The Journal of Clinical Investigation. 2020;**130**(7):3528-3542

[27] Sharma MD et al. Activation of p53 in immature myeloid precursor cells controls differentiation into Ly6c(+)CD103(+) monocytic antigen-presenting cells in tumors. Immunity. 2018;**48**(1):91-106 e6

[28] Kuhn S et al. Increased numbers of monocyte-derived dendritic cells during successful tumor immunotherapy with immune-activating agents. Journal of Immunology. 2013;**191**(4):1984-1992

[29] Kuhn S, Yang J, Ronchese F. Monocyte-derived dendritic cells are essential for CD8(+) T cell activation and antitumor responses after local immunotherapy. Frontiers in Immunology. 2015;**6**:584

[30] Diao J et al. Tumor dendritic cells (DCs) derived from precursors of conventional DCs are dispensable for intratumor CTL responses. Journal of Immunology. 2018;**201**(4):1306-1314

[31] Chow KV et al. Monocyte-derived dendritic cells promote Th polarization, whereas conventional dendritic cells promote Th proliferation. Journal of Immunology. 2016;**196**(2):624-636

[32] Tang-Huau TL et al. Human in vivo-generated monocyte-derived dendritic cells and macrophages cross-present antigens through a vacuolar pathway. Nature Communications. 2018;**9**(1):2570

[33] Wilgenhof S et al. Phase II study of autologous monocyte-derived mRNA electroporated dendritic cells (TriMixDC-MEL) plus ipilimumab in patients with pretreated advanced

melanoma. Journal of Clinical Oncology. 2016;**34**(12):1330-1338

[34] Bol KF et al. Favorable overall survival in stage III melanoma patients after adjuvant dendritic cell vaccination. Oncoimmunology. 2016;**5**(1):e1057673

[35] Rodriguez J et al. A randomized phase II clinical trial of dendritic cell vaccination following complete resection of colon cancer liver metastasis. Journal for Immunotherapy of Cancer. 2018;**6**(1):96

[36] Liau LM et al. First results on survival from a large Phase 3 clinical trial of an autologous dendritic cell vaccine in newly diagnosed glioblastoma. Journal of Translational Medicine. 2018;**16**(1):142

[37] Mastelic-Gavillet B et al. Personalized dendritic cell vaccines-recent breakthroughs and encouraging clinical results. Frontiers in Immunology. 2019;**10**:766

[38] Lavin Y et al. Innate immune landscape in early lung adenocarcinoma by paired single-cell analyses. Cell. 2017;**169**(4):750-765 e17

[39] Wculek SK et al. Dendritic cells in cancer immunology and immunotherapy. Nature Reviews. Immunology. 2020;**20**(1):7-24

[40] Spranger S, Bao R, Gajewski TF. Melanoma-intrinsic beta-catenin signalling prevents anti-tumour immunity. Nature. 2015;**523**(7559):231-235

[41] Ruiz de Galarreta M et al. beta-catenin activation promotes immune escape and resistance to anti-PD-1 therapy in hepatocellular carcinoma. Cancer Discovery. 2019;**9**(8):1124-1141

[42] Wang D, DuBois RN. Role of prostanoids in gastrointestinal cancer. The Journal of Clinical Investigation. 2018;**128**(7):2732-2742

[43] Mizuno R, Kawada K, Sakai Y. Prostaglandin E2/EP signaling in the tumor microenvironment of colorectal cancer. International Journal of Molecular Sciences. 2019;**20**(24):6254

[44] Zelenay S et al. Cyclooxygenase-dependent tumor growth through evasion of immunity. Cell. 2015;**162**(6): 1257-1270

[45] Bonavita E et al. Antagonistic inflammatory phenotypes dictate tumor fate and response to immune checkpoint blockade. Immunity. 2020;**53**(6):1215-1229 e8

[46] Bobr A et al. Autocrine/paracrine TGF-beta1 inhibits Langerhans cell migration. Proceedings of the National Academy of Sciences of the United States of America. 2012;**109**(26):10492-10497

[47] Weber F et al. Transforming growth factor-beta1 immobilises dendritic cells within skin tumours and facilitates tumour escape from the immune system. Cancer Immunology, Immunotherapy. 2005;**54**(9):898-906

[48] Scandella E et al. Prostaglandin E2 is a key factor for CCR7 surface expression and migration of monocyte-derived dendritic cells. Blood. 2002;**100**(4):1354-1361

[49] Diao G et al. Prostaglandin E2 serves a dual role in regulating the migration of dendritic cells. International Journal of Molecular Medicine. 2021;**47**(1):207-218

[50] Amarante-Mendes GP et al. Pattern recognition receptors and the host cell death molecular machinery. Frontiers in Immunology. 2018;**9**:2379

[51] Crotzer VL, Blum JS. Autophagy and adaptive immunity. Immunology. 2010;**131**(1):9-17

[52] Savina A, Amigorena S. Phagocytosis and antigen presentation in dendritic cells. Immunological Reviews. 2007;**219**:143-156

[53] Neefjes J et al. Towards a systems understanding of MHC class I and MHC class II antigen presentation. Nature Reviews. Immunology. 2011;**11**(12):823-836

[54] Lin H et al. Stanniocalcin 1 is a phagocytosis checkpoint driving tumor immune resistance. Cancer Cell. 2021;**39**(4):480-493 e6

[55] Xu F et al. Mevalonate blockade in cancer cells triggers CLEC9A(+) dendritic cell-mediated antitumor immunity. Cancer Research. 2021;**81**(17):4514-4528

[56] Ahrens S et al. F-actin is an evolutionarily conserved damage-associated molecular pattern recognized by DNGR-1, a receptor for dead cells. Immunity. 2012;**36**(4):635-645

[57] Zhang JG et al. The dendritic cell receptor Clec9A binds damaged cells via exposed actin filaments. Immunity. 2012;**36**(4):646-657

[58] de Mingo Pulido A et al. The inhibitory receptor TIM-3 limits activation of the cGAS-STING pathway in intra-tumoral dendritic cells by suppressing extracellular DNA uptake. Immunity. 2021;**54**(6):1154-1167 e7

[59] Baghdadi M et al. TIM-4 glycoprotein-mediated degradation of dying tumor cells by autophagy leads to reduced antigen presentation and increased immune tolerance. Immunity. 2013;**39**(6):1070-1081

[60] Caronni N et al. TIM4 expression by dendritic cells mediates uptake of tumor-associated antigens and anti-tumor responses. Nature Communications. 2021;**12**(1):2237

[61] Herber DL et al. Lipid accumulation and dendritic cell dysfunction in cancer. Nature Medicine. 2010;**16**(8):880-886

[62] Ramakrishnan R et al. Oxidized lipids block antigen cross-presentation by dendritic cells in cancer. Journal of Immunology. 2014;**192**(6):2920-2931

[63] Cubillos-Ruiz JR et al. ER stress sensor XBP1 controls anti-tumor immunity by disrupting dendritic cell homeostasis. Cell. 2015;**161**(7):1527-1538

[64] Veglia F et al. Lipid bodies containing oxidatively truncated lipids block antigen cross-presentation by dendritic cells in cancer. Nature Communications. 2017;**8**(1):2122

[65] Ruffell B et al. Macrophage IL-10 blocks CD8+ T cell-dependent responses to chemotherapy by suppressing IL-12 expression in intratumoral dendritic cells. Cancer Cell. 2014;**26**(5):623-637

[66] Yang L et al. Cancer-associated immunodeficiency and dendritic cell abnormalities mediated by the prostaglandin EP2 receptor. The Journal of Clinical Investigation. 2003;**111**(5):727-735

[67] Liu Q et al. Tumor-educated CD11bhighIalow regulatory dendritic cells suppress T cell response through arginase I. Journal of Immunology. 2009;**182**(10):6207-6216

[68] Scarlett UK et al. Ovarian cancer progression is controlled by phenotypic changes in dendritic cells. The Journal of Experimental Medicine. 2012;**209**(3):495-506

[69] Hanks BA et al. Type III TGF-beta receptor downregulation generates an immunotolerant tumor microenvironment. The Journal of Clinical Investigation. 2013;**123**(9):3925-3940

[70] Terra M et al. Tumor-derived TGFbeta alters the ability of plasmacytoid dendritic cells to respond to innate immune signaling. Cancer Research. 2018;**78**(11):3014-3026

[71] Oussa NA et al. VEGF requires the receptor NRP-1 to inhibit lipopolysaccharide-dependent dendritic cell maturation. Journal of Immunology. 2016;**197**(10):3927-3935

[72] Chae CS et al. Tumor-derived Lysophosphatidic acid blunts protective type-I interferon responses in ovarian cancer. Cancer Discovery. 2022;**12**(8):1904-1921

[73] Raychaudhuri D et al. Lactate induces pro-tumor reprogramming in intratumoral plasmacytoid dendritic cells. Frontiers in Immunology. 2019;**10**:1878

[74] Holtzhausen A et al. Melanoma-derived Wnt5a promotes local dendritic-cell expression of IDO and immunotolerance: Opportunities for pharmacologic enhancement of immunotherapy. Cancer Immunology Research. 2015;**3**(9):1082-1095

[75] Zhao F et al. Paracrine Wnt5a-beta-catenin signaling triggers a metabolic program that drives dendritic cell tolerization. Immunity. 2018;**48**(1):147-160 e7

[76] Kerdidani D et al. Wnt1 silences chemokine genes in dendritic cells and induces adaptive immune resistance in lung adenocarcinoma. Nature Communications. 2019;**10**(1):1405

[77] Fu C et al. beta-catenin in dendritic cells exerts opposite functions in cross-priming and maintenance of CD8+ T cells through regulation of IL-10. Proceedings of the National Academy of Sciences of the United States of America. 2015;**112**(9):2823-2828

[78] Liang X et al. beta-catenin mediates tumor-induced immunosuppression by inhibiting cross-priming of CD8(+) T cells. Journal of Leukocyte Biology. 2014;**95**(1):179-190

[79] Hong Y et al. beta-catenin promotes regulatory T-cell responses in tumors by inducing vitamin A metabolism in dendritic cells. Cancer Research. 2015;**75**(4):656-665

[80] Vander Lugt B et al. Transcriptional determinants of tolerogenic and immunogenic states during dendritic cell maturation. The Journal of Cell Biology. 2017;**216**(3):779-792

[81] Xiao S et al. Retinoic acid increases Foxp3+ regulatory T cells and inhibits development of Th17 cells by enhancing TGF-beta-driven Smad3 signaling and inhibiting IL-6 and IL-23 receptor expression. Journal of Immunology. 2008;**181**(4):2277-2284

[82] Bono MR et al. Retinoic acid as a modulator of T cell immunity. Nutrients. 2016;**8**(6):349

[83] Guilliams M et al. Skin-draining lymph nodes contain dermis-derived CD103(−) dendritic cells that constitutively produce retinoic acid and induce Foxp3(+) regulatory T cells. Blood. 2010;**115**(10):1958-1968

[84] Jiang A et al. Disruption of E-cadherin-mediated adhesion induces a functionally distinct pathway of dendritic cell maturation. Immunity. 2007;**27**(4):610-624

[85] Taniguchi K, Karin M. NF-kappaB, inflammation, immunity and cancer: coming of age. Nature Reviews. Immunology. 2018;**18**(5):309-324

[86] Li R et al. STAT3 and NF-kappaB are simultaneously suppressed in dendritic cells in lung cancer. Scientific Reports. 2017;**7**:45395

[87] Alizadeh D et al. IFNgamma is critical for CAR T cell-mediated myeloid activation and induction of endogenous immunity. Cancer Discovery. 2021;**11**(9):2248-2265

[88] Maier B et al. A conserved dendritic-cell regulatory program limits antitumour immunity. Nature. 2020;**580**(7802):257-262

[89] Ghislat G et al. NF-kappaB-dependent IRF1 activation programs cDC1 dendritic cells to drive antitumor immunity. Science Immunology. 2021;**6**(61):eabg3570

[90] Tas SW et al. Noncanonical NF-kappaB signaling in dendritic cells is required for indoleamine 2,3-dioxygenase (IDO) induction and immune regulation. Blood. 2007;**110**(5):1540-1549

[91] Chiba S et al. Tumor-infiltrating DCs suppress nucleic acid-mediated innate immune responses through interactions between the receptor TIM-3 and the alarmin HMGB1. Nature Immunology. 2012;**13**(9):832-842

[92] de Mingo Pulido A et al. TIM-3 regulates CD103(+) dendritic cell function and response to chemotherapy in breast cancer. Cancer Cell. 2018;**33**(1):60-74 e6

[93] Lee M et al. Immunobiology of nitric oxide and regulation of inducible nitric oxide synthase. Results and Problems in Cell Differentiation. 2017;**62**:181-207

[94] Barilla RM et al. Specialized dendritic cells induce tumor-promoting IL-10(+)IL-17(+) FoxP3(neg) regulatory CD4(+) T cells in pancreatic carcinoma. Nature Communications. 2019;**10**(1):1424

[95] Lawless SJ et al. Glucose represses dendritic cell-induced T cell responses. Nature Communications. 2017;**8**: 15620

[96] Laoui D et al. The tumour microenvironment harbours ontogenically distinct dendritic cell populations with opposing effects on tumour immunity. Nature Communications. 2016;**7**:13720

[97] Croft M, Duncan DD, Swain SL. Response of naive antigen-specific CD4+ T cells in vitro: Characteristics and antigen-presenting cell requirements. The Journal of Experimental Medicine. 1992;**176**(5):1431-1437

[98] Constantino J et al. Dendritic cell-based immunotherapy: A basic review and recent advances. Immunologic Research. 2017;**65**(4):798-810

[99] Draube A et al. Dendritic cell based tumor vaccination in prostate and renal cell cancer: A systematic review and meta-analysis. PLoS One. 2011;**6**(4):e18801

[100] Amos SM et al. Autoimmunity associated with immunotherapy of cancer. Blood. 2011;**118**(3):499-509

[101] Anguille S et al. Clinical use of dendritic cells for cancer therapy. The Lancet Oncology. 2014;**15**(7):e257-e267

[102] Bol KF et al. The clinical application of cancer immunotherapy based on naturally circulating dendritic cells. Journal for Immunotherapy of Cancer. 2019;**7**(1):109

[103] Abraham RS, Mitchell DA. Gene-modified dendritic cell vaccines for cancer. Cytotherapy. 2016;**18**(11): 1446-1455

[104] Perez CR, De Palma M. Engineering dendritic cell vaccines to improve cancer immunotherapy. Nature Communications. 2019;**10**(1):5408

[105] Weller M et al. Rindopepimut with temozolomide for patients with newly diagnosed, EGFRvIII-expressing glioblastoma (ACT IV): A randomised, double-blind, international phase 3 trial. The Lancet Oncology. 2017;**18**(10):1373-1385

[106] Phuphanich S et al. Phase I trial of a multi-epitope-pulsed dendritic cell vaccine for patients with newly diagnosed glioblastoma. Cancer Immunology, Immunotherapy. 2013;**62**(1):125-135

[107] Wen PY et al. A randomized double-blind placebo-controlled phase II trial of dendritic cell vaccine ICT-107 in newly diagnosed patients with glioblastoma. Clinical Cancer Research. 2019;**25**(19):5799-5807

[108] Mitchell DA et al. Tetanus toxoid and CCL3 improve dendritic cell vaccines in mice and glioblastoma patients. Nature. 2015;**519**(7543):366

[109] Batich KA et al. Once, twice, three times a finding: reproducibility of dendritic cell vaccine trials targeting cytomegalovirus in glioblastoma. Clinical Cancer Research. 2020;**26**(20):5297-5303

Chapter 5

Perspective Chapter: Impact of Tumor Metabolism on Immune Cells in the Tumor Microenvironment

Adith Kotha, Chikezie Madu and Yi Lu

Abstract

Metabolism is essential for a cell to obtain energy for its growth and development. In tumors, the rapid rate of cell proliferation leads to an increased demand for energy. Because nutrients in the tumor microenvironment are scarce, there is great competition between tumor cells and healthy cells to obtain them. Because of this, tumor cells undergo adaptations to outcompete healthy cells for nutrients. These adaptations cause characteristic changes to the tumor microenvironment, which in turn, causes changes to immune cells in the tumor tissue. These changes help the tumor evade immune detection and cause tumor growth and metastasis. This review will analyze the changes that take place in the tumor microenvironment, the impact they have on immune cells, and how this contributes to cancer progression.

Keywords: metabolism, nutrients, tumor microenvironment, immune cells, immune detection, cancer progression

1. Introduction

Metabolic reactions are chemical reactions that take place within cells or organisms and are essential for their survival. Metabolic processes include the breakdown of compounds for energy, the synthesis of necessary biomolecules, etc. Changes to the metabolic processes of cancer cells are a key characteristic of tumorigenesis. In order to supply their rapid rates of cell proliferation, tumor cells are in constant need of nutrients from the tumor microenvironment (TME), which are very scarce. This puts tumor cells in fierce competition with neighboring cells for these resources. Tumor cells undergo various adaptations, such as utilizing anaerobic glycolysis in favor of aerobic respiration, a process that allows them to synthesize ATP at higher rates. Such adaptations allow tumor cells to outcompete neighboring cells and allow the tumor to grow. The adaptations that the tumor cells undergo have an influence on the TME. For example, the aforementioned use of anaerobic respiration causes the TME to become more hypoxic and acidic.

These changes to the characteristics of the TME cause phenotypic alterations of immune cells within the TME. The TME includes cells of both the adaptive and innate immune systems, and they undergo notable changes to their metabolic pathways in response to the conditions of the TME or other signals within it. The former includes T cells and B cells, while the latter consists of tumor-associated macrophages (TAMs), natural killer (NK) cells, dendritic cells, and neutrophils.

These alterations of immune cells in the TME provide numerous benefits to the tumor. Namely, various altered pathways allow for the tumor to evade detection by the immune system, which contributes to the growth of tumors and the progression of cancer. This paper will discuss how the metabolic reprogramming of tumor cells contributes to changes in the conditions of the TME, the impact these changes have on the functionality of immune cells, and how they relate to the spread of cancer.

2. Changes to conditions of the TME

Tumor growth relies on the rapid proliferation of cells, which is an energetically demanding process. However, nutrients within the TME are often very scarce, and as a result, tumor cells are in fierce competition with healthy cells in the TME for these nutrients. Tumor cells adapt to these increased energy demands by shifting their metabolic pathways [1]. One such adaptation that tumor cells undergo is reprogramming of their glucose metabolism to utilize anaerobic glycolysis in preference to the tricarboxylic (TCA) and oxidative phosphorylation (OXPHOS) pathways ([2], **Figure 1**). This pathway, known as the Warburg effect, is active even in the presence of abundant oxygen, and it is key to a tumor cell's ability to outcompete neighboring cells.

Though the process of anaerobic glycolysis generates lower quantities of net ATP from glucose than the OXPHOS pathway, it allows for the metabolism of glucose to occur much more rapidly in tumor cells, thus leading to tumor cells outcompeting neighboring ones for nutrients. Additionally, other adaptive mechanisms of tumor

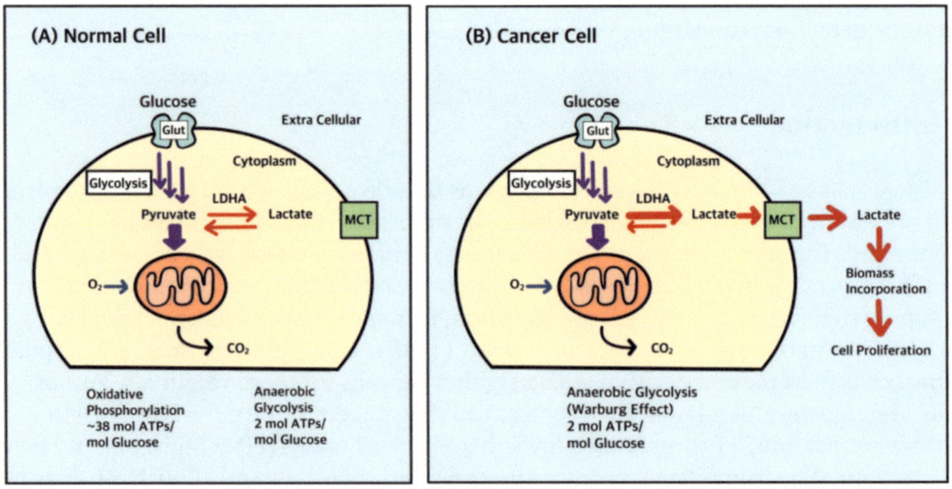

Figure 1.
(Warburg effect): The Warburg effect is a major metabolic reprogramming that cancer cells undergo. Normal cells exhibit a usage of both glycolytic and OXPHOS pathways, while cancer cells rely on glycolysis and produce excess lactate as a by-product. This reliance on glycolysis and production of molecules, such as lactate, cause major changes to the conditions of the TME [3].

cells allow them to overcome this inefficient method of obtaining energy. For example, many tumor cells can carry out autophagy, which allows them to recycle nutrients and prevents nutrient depletion [4]. Additionally, tumor cells can synthesize ATP using two ADP molecules, forming one ATP and one AMP [5, 6]. These adaptations make the Warburg effect a useful mechanism through which tumor cells can outcompete other cells within the TME for nutrients and proliferate. However, the process also causes drastic changes to the conditions of the TME.

The primary change caused by the Warburg effect is the acidification of the TME. These conditions are caused by the higher rates of anaerobic glycolysis and the production of lactic acid [7]. The acidic state of the TME confers numerous advantages for tumor growth, as it promotes the formation of new blood vessels, drug resistance, and suppression of the anticancer immune system [8]. The lactic acid that is produced can also act as a signaling molecule that regulates the migration of tumor cells: areas with a lower pH promote tumor cell invasion and metastasis [8].

Another important characteristic of the TME is its state of hypoxia. The delivery of oxygen and other nutrients to tissue occurs through blood vessels. Because tumors are undergoing constant growth, their receiving of blood flow is often irregular. In order to combat this, tumor tissues can form new blood vessels in a process referred to as angiogenesis [9]. This process allows tumors to continually receive the nutrients required to meet their metabolic demands. However, if angiogenesis fails, the aforementioned conditions of hypoxia and resource scarcity will arise in the TME. The tumor can still thrive under these conditions due to its reliance on anaerobic glycolysis [7]. Additionally, the hypoxic state acts as an additional stressor on the immune system and allows the tumor to evade immune attack.

The conditions in the TME also cause changes to the functionality of the immune system. For example, the hypoxic environment can negatively impact the immune detection of cancer cells and contributes to tumor immunity [10]. Signaling factors, called hypoxia-inducible factors (HIFs), are a key part of the regulation of tumor immunity genes. These factors can also inactivate lymphocytes in the TME, namely NK cells and CD8 T lymphocytes, thus preventing them from combating tumor growth. In this pathway, proinflammatory signals produced in hypoxic regions of the TME attract regulatory T cells (Tregs), which in turn suppress cytotoxic T cells from producing an immune response, thus promoting cancer growth [11]. The hypoxic conditions also act as a stressor on neutrophils and block them from attacking tumors. Finally, HIFs have negative impacts on the maturation of B cells, which they accomplish by increasing their rate of glycolysis. This metabolic change to B cells causes them to divide less rapidly (thus decreasing their immune response), prevents them from altering antibody production, and can even trigger cell death [10].

Additionally, the aerobic glycolysis pathway causes irregularities in the metabolite balance within tumor cells, a factor that causes changes to cell signaling and cell–cell interactions within the TME [12]. For example, the aforementioned acidic conditions of the TME created by the excessive lactate produced through glycolytic pathways interfere with the immune response of cytotoxic T cells. The lactic acid also interferes with the production of IFN-γ by NK cells, which inhibits phagocytic cells from attacking the tumor [13].

Amino acids, namely glutamine, arginine, and tryptophan, are also important metabolites that influence the function of immune cells within the TME. Glutamine is produced as a by-product of the catabolism of proteins in nutrient-scarce environments [13]. It is essential to the function of immune cells because it regulates immune cell activation and determination, namely that of T cells. When its availability is limited, T-cell functionality is suppressed [13]. Similar to glutamine, arginine plays a role in the activation of T cells and NK cells. Additionally, it regulates the secretion of cytokines [13]. Tumor cells consume a significant amount of the exogenous arginine in the TME, thus inhibiting the effect it has on immune cells [13]. Tryptophan also plays a role in the regulation of T cells, namely its cell cycle. When tryptophan is unavailable, the rate of T-cell apoptosis increases drastically [13].

Finally, lipids play an important role in the regulation of immune cell signaling within the TME. Fatty acids are needed for macrophage maturation and proliferation [13]. Additionally, they are necessary for the synthesis of membranes for effector immune cells. However, the accumulation of fatty acids within the TME can cause metabolic alterations to immune cells and make them anti-inflammatory. [13]. Similar effects can be induced by the accumulation of cholesterol within the TME, which causes T cells to lose their antitumor functionality. This occurs because high cholesterol levels can cause the disruption of T-cell membranes, thus impeding their ability to attack tumors [13].

3. Immune cell subtypes in TME

The tumor microenvironment is comprised of tumor cells, resident host cells, extracellular matrix, cancer-associated fibroblasts, vascular cells, and tumor-infiltrating immune cells [14]. Although tumor-infiltrating immune cells of both innate and adaptive arms of the immune system are often present in the TME, specific subtypes of immune cells, their number, and function can vary significantly depending on the tumor type and on the different stages of progression [14]. Functionally, tumor-infiltrating immune cells have been shown to be responsible for both tumor-inhibitory (antitumor) and tumor-promoting properties [15]. Recruitment of immune cells into the TME is tightly regulated by chemotactic factors and the expression of chemokine receptors on immune cells which together define the recruitment of activator or suppressor type of immune cells into the TME [16]. Based on the extent of immune cell infiltration into tumor tissue, the TME can be classified as immune-infiltrated, immune-excluded, and immune-silent.

Immune cells of the adaptive response in the TME include T- and B- subsets of lymphocytes. Both subtypes of CD3+ T lymphocytes (CD4+ helper T cells and CD8+ cytotoxic T cells) can be observed within the TME, where CD8+ T cells are predominantly responsible for cytotoxicity response against the tumor cells and CD4+ T cells either support CD8+ cell cytotoxic activity or act as regulatory T cells (Tregs) that suppress the antitumor immune responses. The types of chemotactic factors in the TME and expression cytokine receptors therefore collectively determine which subtype of T cells predominate in the TME. For example, chemokines CXCR3, and CXCR4 aid in directing the migration of cytotoxic T cells and NK cells into the tumor, whereas CCR4 expression is linked to the recruitment of suppressor Tregs into the TME [16]. B cells, which are primarily responsible for antibody-mediated immune response, are also observed in the TME but in relatively small numbers when compared with T cells. Tumor-infiltrating B cells appear to mediate the formation of lymphoid-like structures within the TME where their interaction with T cells regulates tumor progression [16].

Immune cells of innate response that are constituents of the TME include NK cells, macrophages, neutrophils, and dendritic cells [14, 16]. Natural killer (NK cells) mediate antitumor activity either via direct cell-mediated killing of tumor cells or by secretion of specific cytokines that indirectly contribute to the antitumor response. NK cells, although present in the TME, are less efficient at killing tumor cells within the tumor microenvironment, are highly effective against circulating tumor cells, and therefore more effective in preventing tumor metastasis [17]. Macrophages by far are the most common type of innate immune cells in TME and macrophage infiltration has been associated with poor prognosis of several solid tumors. Two distinct phenotypes of macrophages that mediate a pro-inflammatory response (M1 macrophages) and wound healing response (M2 macrophages) are commonly present in the tumor tissue [18]. However, the hypoxic state and presence of certain cytokines within the TME favor the M2 phenotype that supports tumor progression [18]. Neutrophils are the next variety of innate immune cells seen in the TME. Neutrophils are recruited into tumor tissue where they initially promote a local inflammatory response thereby promoting tumor cell apoptosis. As the tumor progresses, neutrophils can functionally support tumor growth through the modification of the extracellular matrix, and the release of growth factors that promote angiogenesis [19]. Dendritic cells (DCs), the most potent type of antigen-presenting cells; play an important role in cancer immunosurveillance and infiltration of DC into tumor tissue is associated with delayed tumor progression and metastasis [19].

4. Metabolism in lymphocytes: t cells

Metabolic pathways in T-lymphocyte vary depending on their differentiation status in their life cycle [20]. Naïve T lymphocytes mainly depend on TCA and OXPHOS to support basal metabolism. Continued signaling from cytokines, such as IL-7, is required to maintain glucose uptake by naïve T cells for sustaining the metabolism [20]. Following antigen recognition and activation, T cells undergo a metabolic change that is dependent on both glucose and amino acids as energy sources to support cell proliferation and to function as effector T cells [21]. Similar to the tumor cells, the effector T cells use Warburg metabolism to support energy demands associated with the secretion of cytotoxic cytokines and enzymes required for the removal of the tumor and virally infected cells. Therefore, within the TME, malignant cells compete with the effector T cells for energy sources and relatively nutrient deficiency in the TME can impair T-cell survival and proliferation [22]. The mechanisms underlying the regulation of T-cell effector functions by metabolic pathways also vary in different subsets of T cells. For example, in CD4 T cells, enzymes of the glycolytic pathway, such as GAPDH, can interact with mRNA of key cytokines, thereby preventing their translation [23]. Additionally, acetyl-CoA produced from citrate in cytosol due to the action of ATP citrate lyase (ACL) in both CD4 and CD8 T cells can directly modify histone acetylation status at the promoter regions of key cytokine genes involved in mediating effector functions [24]. Changes in mitochondrial structure and function are also implicated in the regulation of effector T-cell function as well as memory T-cell formation. Effector T cells, where mitochondria exhibit fragmentation, are poor in supporting electron transport machinery that leads to upregulation of anaerobic glycolysis, whereas in memory T cells, the mitochondrial fusion process allows proper function of ETC and facilitates lipid metabolism via fatty acid oxidation [25].

Due to similarities in the metabolic pathways utilized, within the TME, competition for nutrients exists between tumor cells and the effector T cells [26]. Tumor cells with functional mutations that confer survival advantage can therefore outcompete effector T cells leading to the reduced number and/or function of cytotoxic CD8 cells. Furthermore, lactate produced by tumor cells in the hypoxic regions creates an acidic environment that can inhibit T-cell activation by preventing glycolysis [27]. In contrast with cytotoxic T cells, Tregs, upon activation, induce fatty acid biosynthesis and oxidative phosphorylation, conferring them with a metabolic advantage to thrive within the TME [28]. Tumor cells evade the immune response by upregulation of inhibitory receptors, such as programmed cell death protein 1 (PD-1) and cytotoxic T-lymphocyte association protein 4 (CTLA4). These inhibitory receptors, known as immune checkpoints, are widely used as targets in cancer therapy as they also play a role in the metabolic regulation of T cells [29]. PD-1 expression downregulates glycolysis and increases fatty acid oxidation, which reduces their cytotoxic potential. PD-L1 expressed on tumor cells enhances glucose uptake and therefore blockade of PD-1/PD-L1 interaction can collectively potentiate antitumor activity of T cells [30]. CTLA-4 is a receptor expressed transiently on T cells following activation and plays an important role in regulating their activity. One of the mechanisms by which CTLA-4 suppresses T-cell activity is by down-regulating critical amino acid and nutrient transporters and inhibition of CTLA4 can restore the bioenergetic balance that favors the survival of T cells in the TME [29].

Another key area where understanding T-cell metabolism is critical is in cell-based therapies that utilize chimeric antigen receptor (CAR)-T and tumor-infiltrating lymphocytes (TIL). CAR-T treatment is an immunotherapeutic strategy in which samples of T cells taken from a patient's blood are genetically modified to produce receptors that target tumor cells [31]. In TIL therapy, T lymphocytes are taken from the tumor microenvironment and cultured *ex vivo*. The amplified TILs are then infused with the tumor in order to promote the targeting of cancer cells. These cells undergo metabolic reprogramming to inhibit glycolysis *in vivo*, which increases the

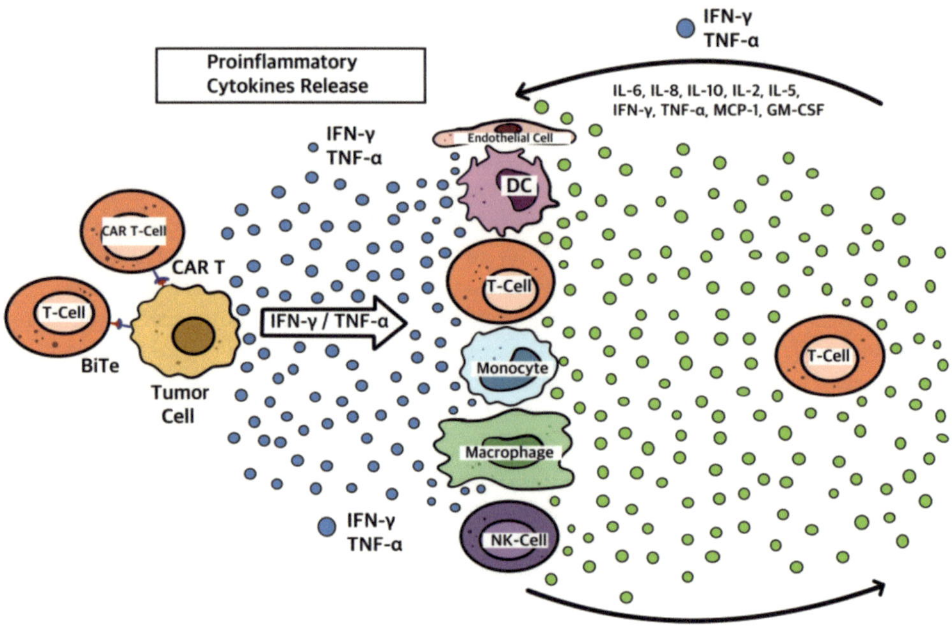

Figure 2.
(cytokine release syndrome): CRS is an acute immune inflammatory response caused by the activation of the immune system, particularly T cells. This triggers the release of cytokines, which are molecules involved in directing immune function. These excess cytokines pose serious health risks, such as organ failure and potential death [34].

proliferation of T cells and thus increases antitumor efficacy [32]. These methods have proven beneficial as alternative therapies when conventional therapies fail due to the acquisition of tumor resistance or where checkpoint inhibitors therapies are not a viable option due to lack of expression of those receptors as targets [33]. Both CAR-T and TIL therapies require isolation and *ex vivo* expansion of tumor-specific lymphocytes prior to administering to the patients. Despite having tumor-specific activity, engineered CAR-T-cell therapies are prone to adverse events in the form of cytokine release syndrome ([32], **Figure 2**). It is beginning to be understood that some of the mechanisms underlying CAR-T-cell properties, therapeutic efficacy, and potential adverse events are linked to metabolic pathways in the engineered cells. Conditions used for *ex vivo* expansion of TIL and CAR-T cells also may alter the metabolic state of these cells, thus impacting therapeutic effectiveness [35]. It is possible that redirecting the metabolic pathways during their expansion may result in cells with beneficial properties targeting tumors [35].

5. Metabolism in lymphocytes: nk cells

Resting NK cells predominately use glucose as fuel to carry out glycolysis and oxidative phosphorylation. Activation of NK cells via cytokine stimulation increases glucose uptake and the rate of glycolysis and oxidative phosphorylation, which support biosynthesis and secretion of IFN-Y and other key enzymes, such as granzyme, that are required for NK cell effector function [35]. In contrast with other lymphocytes, pyruvate generated from glycolysis in NK cells is preferentially converted to citrate via citrate-malate shuttle (CMS) rather than metabolism via the TCA cycle [36]. Two subsets of NK cells are recognized based on the expression level of phenotypic marker CD56 (CD56 dim and CD56 bright) that appear to be metabolically distinct. For example, CD56 bright NK cells involved in cytokine production express higher levels of glucose transporter proteins, thus rapidly taking up glucose upon activation [37]. In addition to glucose, glutamine is also important as a fuel source for the metabolism of activated NK cells. Glutamine can regulate the uptake of critical amino acids and the breakdown products of glutamine enter the TCA cycle for generating ATP [37]. Metabolic pathways in NK cells are tightly regulated both during development and activation. Specific signal transduction pathways and transcription factors are involved in regulating the metabolic pathways in NK cells. Transcription factor steroid regulatory element binding protein (SREBP) regulates the expression of the components of the CMS pathway and the mammalian target of the rapamycin (mTOR) pathway regulates NK cell proliferation and metabolism [36]. Consequently, reduced mTOR activity of mature NK cells is associated with diminished metabolic activity that results in impaired effector functions of NK cells. The multifunctional transcription factor c-Myc plays an important role by upregulating glucose transporters and critical enzymes of glycolysis in NK cells [36].

Although NK cells are highly effective in the targeted removal of tumor cells, the tumor microenvironment poses a challenge to the appropriate function of the NK cells. Firstly, changes in the metabolic properties of tumor cells create an environment that is low in critical nutrients (glucose and glutamine) and oxygen (hypoxic state) that are essential for the normal metabolism of NK cells [38]. Secondly, anaerobic glycolysis of tumor cells produces lactic acid that creates an unfavorable acidic environment, leading to reactive oxygen species (ROS) production in NK cells and induction of apoptosis [38]. Furthermore, transforming growth factor β

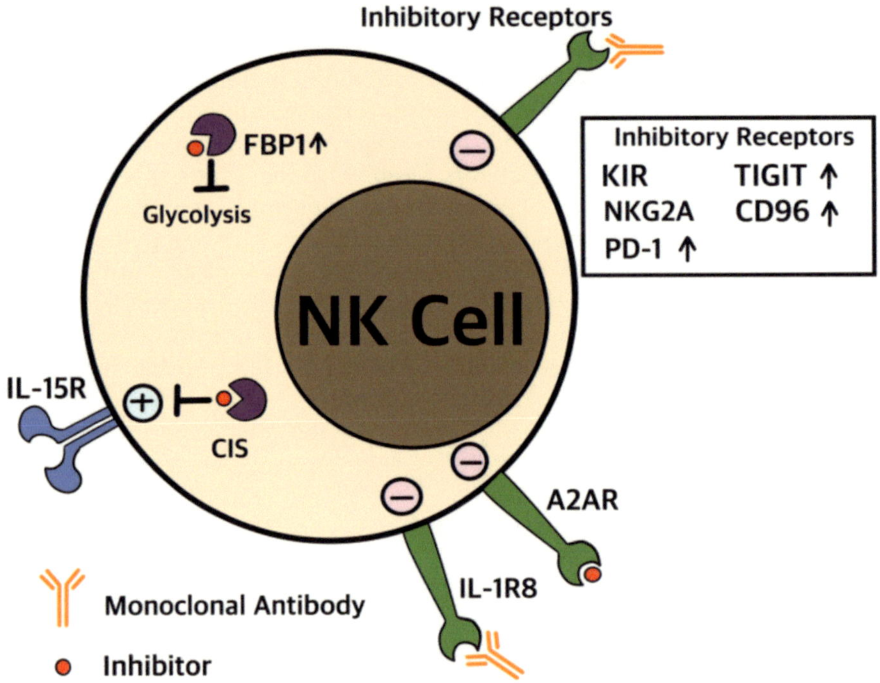

Figure 3.
(targeting of NK-cell metabolic pathways): The targeting of major receptors and metabolites, namely FBP-1 in NK cells, holds great promise in restoring the antitumor efficacy of NK cells in the TME [40].

(TGF-β), a cytokine that is commonly upregulated in several cancers can inhibit NK cell metabolism, presumably via the inhibition of mTor activity [39]. Metabolic adaptation of NK cells within the TME involves the activation of enzymes in the gluconeogenetic pathways, such as FBP-1, to generate glucose needed for NK cell metabolism. Therefore, dysregulated FBP-1 expression in NK cells further reduces their ability to survive in the TME and thus reduces immune function [40]. The hypoxic state of TME is associated with mitochondrial fragmentation in certain tumors, which perturb the survival and cytotoxic properties of NK cells [41]. In addition to the aforementioned factors, certain other metabolites that are elevated in the TME (adenosine, prostaglandin E2 (PGE2), and kynurenine) may also be responsible for reduced NK cell function via mechanisms that are yet to be understood [36]. Restoring normal metabolic function and survival of NK cells in the TME is one of the bases for pharmacological approaches to treat cancer where infiltrated NK cells have potent antitumor activity. Targeting TGF-β or its downstream signaling pathways and/or restoration of c-Myc protein levels via inhibition of enzymes (GSK3) are potential therapeutic approaches [39]. Additionally, culturing autologous NK cells *ex vivo* and inhibiting FBP-1 has proven to restore immune function, namely cytotoxicity ([40], **Figure 3**). Other cells in the TME (cytotoxic and Tregs, stromal fibroblasts, etc.) have also been shown to modulate the expression of various activating and inhibitory receptors on NK cells that in turn regulate the metabolic and antitumor properties of NK cells [38]. Therefore, targeting inhibitory NK cell receptors, such as NKG2A, is one of the strategies being evaluated as NK cell-mediated antitumor immunotherapy ([38], **Figure 3**).

6. Metabolism in the innate immune system: tumor-associated macrophages

Macrophages are specialized immune cells that develop from myeloid progenitor cells and are highly efficient in phagocytosis and the removal of pathogens [42]. Tumor-associated macrophages (TAMs) are macrophages that are specifically recruited into tumor tissue due to cytokines and growth factors secreted by cells within the tumor microenvironment [43]. TAMs are one of the most abundant leukocytes within the TME and have been implicated in tumor progression and metastasis [44]. Macrophages were further classified as inactive (M0), pro-inflammatory (M1), and anti-inflammatory (M2) subtypes based on specific immune responses elicited by these cells. Inactive macrophages (M0) are undifferentiated cells and can reprogram themselves into polarized M1 and M2 cells after exposure to stimuli [45]. These distinct subtypes of macrophages utilize different metabolic pathways to exert their functional effects and TAMs are further induced to undergo a metabolic switch to survive in the tumor microenvironment. The key features of M1 and M2 macrophages in the utilization of various metabolic pathways are as follows. Although both M1 and M2 macrophages metabolize glucose via glycolytic pathways, in M1 macrophages it is essential for pro-inflammatory properties, such as cytokine production, and in mediating phagocytosis [46]. Similarly, the pentose phosphate pathway, which produces NADPH, is also critical in M1 macrophages, where NADPH-oxidase-dependent generation of reactive oxygen species (ROS) and regeneration of glutathione [47]. Arginine is also metabolized differently in M1 and M2 macrophages by virtue of the

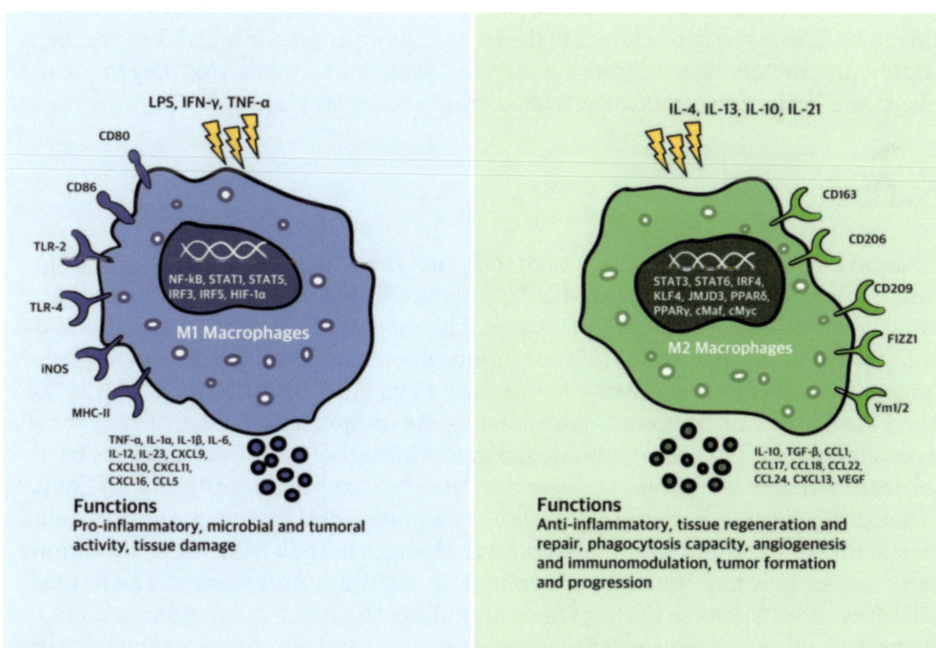

Figure 4.
(TAM polarization): TAMs undergo metabolic changes that trigger polarization to the M2 phenotype, which has pro-tumorigenic properties and contributes to cancer progression [51].

expression of distinct enzymes that break down arginine. Notably, M1 cells express inducible nitric oxide Synthase or iNOs that produces NO from arginine [46] and M2 macrophages express the enzyme arginase that metabolizes arginine to produce ornithine. NO has an important function in mediating pro-inflammatory response and ornithine serves as a precursor for polyamine synthesis that is critical in wound healing and repair processes that are mediated by M2 macrophages [48]. The TCA cycle in M2 macrophages is coupled to mitochondrial oxidative phosphorylation, whereas in M1 macrophages, intermediate metabolites of the TCA cycle, citrate and succinate, accumulate and are redirected toward the processes that lead to the production of inflammatory mediators, such as prostaglandin E2 (PGE2) [49].

The subtypes of macrophages within the TME vary with the progression of tumors. During the early stages of tumors, M1 macrophage polarization is favored, thus leading to the recruitment of cytotoxic CD8 cells and NK cells ([50], **Figure 4**) and the antitumor property of TAMs. However, as tumors progress, polarization to M2 macrophages is favored due to progressive changes in the TME ([50], **Figure 4**). Due to aerobic glycolysis of tumor cells, lactic acid in the TME induces M2-like TAM polarization of TAMs [46]. Additionally, TAMs have also been implicated in regulating tumor metastasis and angiogenesis further supporting the survival and spread of tumors. Metabolically, TAMs utilize glucose as the primary energy source with oxidative phosphorylation favoring their differentiation into pro-tumorogenic M2 macrophages [46]. As TAMs constitute the predominant cell population in the TME, potential therapies for cancer are based on metabolic targeting either to inhibit TAM polarization to an M2 phenotype or to selectively deplete M2 cells within the TME [52]. However, considering the complexity of concurrent metabolic processes occurring in other cells in the TME, these approaches have some limitations. Nevertheless, inhibition of OXPHOS pathways in TAMs has been shown to decrease tumor progression [53]. Future therapies directing metabolic processes via targeted drug delivery to TAMs may prove useful to overcome limitations associated with current strategies [52].

7. Conclusion

Cancer cells undergo key changes to their metabolic processes as an adaptation to outcompete other cells in the TME. This metabolic reprogramming causes the chemical conditions of the TME to change. The most notable of these changes is the development of hypoxic and acidic conditions due to a reliance on anaerobic glycolysis rather than OXPHOS pathways to produce ATP (Warburg effect), as well as the limited availability of nutrients. Additionally, the unique metabolism of cancer cells causes irregularities in the metabolite balance within the TME. Such changes have significant impacts on immune cells within the TME and their antitumor efficacy. All immune cell types in the TME of both the adaptive and innate immune systems undergo metabolic alterations in response to changes in the TME. These alterations greatly reduce immune function and contribute to tumor progression. The limited availability of nutrients in the TME downregulates the function of effector T cells and cytotoxic T cells and prevent their proliferation, and also prevents the formation of memory T cells. The antitumor efficacy of NK cells is reduced by the acidic and nutrient-scarce TME, which both triggers apoptosis, as well as the hypoxic state, which triggers mitochondrial fragmentation and reduces cytotoxic capabilities. The conditions of the TME cause TAMs to undergo polarization to the M2 subtype, which has pro-tumorigenic properties and can contribute to angiogenesis. Metabolism in the TME has become a focus of cancer treatment. Common treatments are based on culturing autologous immune cell types *ex vivo* and modifying their metabolic properties. These immune cells are amplified in order to improve immune function and are then infused with the tumor. These treatments must be further explored, but the targeting of immune cell metabolism in the TME proves to be a promising strategy in the treatment of cancer.

Acknowledgements

Funding for the publication of this paper was made possible by a grant from the Assisi Foundation of Memphis. Brown, Chester, PhD (PI). We also thank Yirui Tang for drawing the figures used in this paper.

Conflict of interest

The authors have declared that no conflict of interest exists.

Author details

Adith Kotha[1], Chikezie Madu[1,2] and Yi Lu[3*]

1 Department of Biology, White Station High School, Memphis, USA

2 Department of Biological Sciences, University of Memphis, Memphis, USA

3 Department of Pathology and Laboratory Medicine, University of Tennessee Health Science Center, Memphis, USA

*Address all correspondence to: ylu@utshc.edu

References

[1] Gupta S, Roy A, Dwarakanath BS. Metabolic cooperation and competition in the tumor microenvironment: Implications for therapy. Frontiers in Oncology. 2017;7:68. DOI: 10.3389/fonc.2017.00068

[2] Reina-Campos M, Moscat J, Diaz-Meco M. Metabolism shapes the tumor microenvironment. Current Opinion in Cell Biology. 2017;**48**:47-53. DOI: 10.1016/j.ceb.2017.05.006

[3] Kim, S.-H., & Baek, K.-H. (2021). Regulation of cancer metabolism by deubiquitinating enzymes: The Warburg effect. International Journal of Molecular Sciences, 22(12), 6173. Retrieved from: DOI: 10.3390/ijms22126173

[4] Yang X, Yu DD, Yan F, et al. The role of autophagy induced by tumor microenvironment in different cells and stages of cancer. Cell & Bioscience. 2015;**5**:14. DOI: 10.1186/s13578-015-0005-2

[5] Baghban R, Roshangar L, Jahanban-Esfahlan R, Seidi K, Ebrahimi-Kalan A, Jaymand M, et al. Tumor microenvironment complexity and therapeutic implications at a glance. Cell Communication and Signaling: CCS. 2020;**18**(1):59. DOI: 10.1186/s12964-020-0530-4

[6] Vander Heiden MG, Cantley LC, Thompson CB. Understanding the Warburg effect: The metabolic requirements of cell proliferation. Science. 2009;**324**(5930):1029-1033. DOI: 10.1126/science.1160809

[7] Liberti MV, Locasale JW. The Warburg effect: How does it benefit cancer cells? Trends in Biochemical Sciences. 2016;**41**(3):211-218. DOI: 10.1016/j.tibs.2015.12.001

[8] Wang JX, Choi S, Niu X, Kang N, Xue H, Killam J, et al. Lactic acid and an acidic tumor microenvironment suppress anticancer immunity. International Journal of Molecular Sciences. 2020;**21**(21):8363. DOI: 10.3390/ijms21218363

[9] Nagy JA, Chang SH, Dvorak AM, Dvorak HF. Why are tumour blood vessels abnormal and why is it important to know? British Journal of Cancer. 2009;**100**(6):865-869. DOI: 10.1038/sj.bjc.6604929

[10] Li Y, Zhao L, Li XF. Hypoxia and the tumor microenvironment. Technology in Cancer Research & Treatment. 2021;**20**:15330338211036304. DOI: 10.1177/15330338211036304

[11] Verma NK, Wong B, Poh ZS, Udayakumar A, Verma R, Goh R, et al. Obstacles for T-lymphocytes in the tumour microenvironment: Therapeutic challenges, advances and opportunities beyond immune checkpoint. eBioMedicine. 2022;**83**:104216 Advance online publication. DOI: 10.1016/j.ebiom.2022.104216

[12] Elia I, Haigis MC. Metabolites and the tumour microenvironment: From cellular mechanisms to systemic metabolism. Nature Metabolism. 2021;**3**(1):21-32. DOI: 10.1038/s42255-020-00317-z

[13] Xia L, Oyang L, Lin J, et al. The cancer metabolic reprogramming and immune response. Molecular Cancer. 2021;**20**:28. DOI: 10.1186/s12943-021-01316-8

[14] Anderson NM, Simon MC. The tumor microenvironment. Current Biology: CB. 2020;**30**(16):R921-R925. DOI: 10.1016/j.cub.2020.06.081

[15] Gajewski TF, Schreiber H, Fu YX. Innate and adaptive immune cells in

the tumor microenvironment. Nature Immunology. 2013;**14**(10):1014-1022. DOI: 10.1038/ni.2703

[16] Kohli K, Pillarisetty VG, Kim TS. Key chemokines direct migration of immune cells in solid tumors. Cancer Gene Therapy. 2022;**29**(1):10-21. DOI: 10.1038/s41417-021-00303-x

[17] Terrén I, Orrantia A, Vitallé J, Zenarruzabeitia O, Borrego F. NK cell metabolism and tumor microenvironment. Frontiers in Immunology. 2019;**10**:2278. DOI: 10.3389/fimmu.2019.02278

[18] Mehla K, Singh PK. Metabolic regulation of macrophage polarization in cancer. Trends in Cancer. 2019;**5**(12):822-834. DOI: 10.1016/j.trecan.2019.10.007

[19] Hinshaw DC, Shevde LA. The tumor microenvironment innately modulates cancer progression. Cancer Research. 2019;**79**(18):4557-4566. DOI: 10.1158/0008-5472.CAN-18-3962

[20] Gerriets VA, Rathmell JC. Metabolic pathways in T cell fate and function. Trends in Immunology. 2012;**33**(4):168-173. DOI: 10.1016/j.it.2012.01.010

[21] van der Windt GJ, Pearce EL. Metabolic switching and fuel choice during T-cell differentiation and memory development. Immunological Reviews. 2012;**249**(1):27-42. DOI: 10.1111/j.1600-065X.2012.01150.x

[22] Anderson KG, Stromnes IM, Greenberg PD. Obstacles posed by the tumor microenvironment to T cell activity: A case for synergistic therapies. Cancer Cell. 2017;**31**(3):311-325. DOI: 10.1016/j.ccell.2017.02.008

[23] Bishop EL, Gudgeon N, Dimeloe S. Control of T cell metabolism by cytokines and hormones. Frontiers in Immunology. 2021;**12**:653605. DOI: 10.3389/fimmu.2021.653605

[24] Dominguez M, Brüne B, Namgaladze D. Exploring the role of ATP-citrate lyase in the immune system. Frontiers in Immunology. 2021;**12**: 632526. DOI: 10.3389/fimmu.2021.632526

[25] Geltink R, Kyle RL, Pearce EL. Unraveling the complex interplay between T cell metabolism and function. Annual Review of Immunology. 2018;**36**:461-488. DOI: 10.1146/annurev-immunol-042617-053019

[26] Chang CH, Qiu J, O'Sullivan D, Buck MD, Noguchi T, Curtis JD, et al. Metabolic competition in the tumor microenvironment is a driver of cancer progression. Cell. 2015;**162**(6):1229-1241. DOI: 10.1016/j.cell.2015.08.016

[27] Lim AR, Rathmell WK, Rathmell JC. The tumor microenvironment as a metabolic barrier to effector T cells and immunotherapy. eLife. 2020;**9**:e55185. DOI: 10.7554/eLife.55185

[28] Aristin Revilla S, Kranenburg O, Coffer PJ. Colorectal cancer-infiltrating regulatory t cells: functional heterogeneity, metabolic adaptation, and therapeutic targeting. Frontiers in Immunology. 2022;**13**:903564. DOI: 10.3389/fimmu.2022.903564

[29] Tsai HF, Hsu PN. Cancer immunotherapy by targeting immune checkpoints: mechanism of T cell dysfunction in cancer immunity and new therapeutic targets. Journal of Biomedical Science. 2017;**24**(1):35. DOI: 10.1186/s12929-017-0341-0

[30] Blank C, Gajewski TF, Mackensen A. Interaction of PD-L1 on tumor cells with PD-1 on tumor-specific T cells as a mechanism of immune evasion: implications for tumor immunotherapy. Cancer Immunology, Immunotherapy: CII. 2005;**54**(4):307-314. DOI: 10.1007/s00262-004-0593-x

[31] Siegler EL, Kenderian SS. Neurotoxicity and cytokine release syndrome after chimeric antigen receptor T cell therapy: Insights into mechanisms and novel therapies. Frontiers in Immunology. 2020;**11**:1973. DOI: 10.3389/fimmu.2020.01973

[32] Wu R, Forget MA, Chacon J, Bernatchez C, Haymaker C, Chen JQ, et al. Adoptive T-cell therapy using autologous tumor-infiltrating lymphocytes for metastatic melanoma: Current status and future outlook. Cancer Journal. 2012;**18**(2):160-175. DOI: 10.1097/ppo.0b013e31824d4465

[33] Darvin P, Toor SM, Sasidharan Nair V, Elkord E. Immune checkpoint inhibitors: recent progress and potential biomarkers. Experimental & Molecular Medicine. 2018;**50**(12):1-11. DOI: 10.1038/s12276-018-0191-1

[34] Cosenza M, Sacchi S, Pozzi S. Cytokine release syndrome associated with T-cell-based therapies for hematological malignancies: pathophysiology, clinical presentation, and treatment. International Journal of Molecular Sciences. 2021;**22**(14):7652. Retrieved from:. DOI: 10.3390/ijms22147652

[35] Keppel MP, Saucier N, Mah AY, Vogel TP, Cooper MA. Activation-specific metabolic requirements for NK Cell IFN-γ production. Journal of Immunology. 2015, 1950;**194**(4):1954-1962. DOI: 10.4049/jimmunol.1402099

[36] Cong J. Metabolism of natural killer cells and other innate lymphoid cells. Frontiers in Immunology. 2020;**11**:1989. DOI: 10.3389/fimmu.2020.01989

[37] Mah AY, Cooper MA. Metabolic regulation of natural killer cell IFN-γ production. Critical Reviews in Immunology. 2016;**36**(2):131-147. DOI: 10.1615/CritRevImmunol.2016017387

[38] Domagala J, Lachota M, Klopotowska M, Graczyk-Jarzynka A, Domagala A, Zhylko A, et al. The tumor microenvironment-A metabolic obstacle to NK cells' activity. Cancers. 2020;**12**(12):3542. DOI: 10.3390/cancers12123542

[39] Regis S, Dondero A, Caliendo F, Bottino C, Castriconi R. NK cell function regulation by TGF-β-induced epigenetic mechanisms. Frontiers in Immunology. 2020;**11**:311. DOI: 10.3389/fimmu.2020.00311

[40] Bi J, Tian Z. NK cell dysfunction and checkpoint immunotherapy. Frontiers in Immunology. 2019;**10**:1999. DOI: 10.3389/fimmu.2019.01999

[41] Zheng X, Qian Y, Fu B, Jiao D, Jiang Y, Chen P, et al. Mitochondrial fragmentation limits NK cell-based tumor immunosurveillance. Nature Immunology. 2019;**20**(12):1656-1667. DOI: 10.1038/s41590-019-0511-1

[42] Myeloid-derived suppressor Cells. Linking inflammation and cancer suzanne Ostrand-Rosenberg, Pratima Sinha. The Journal of Immunology. 2009;**182**(8):4499-4506. DOI: 10.4049/jimmunol.0802740

[43] Zhou J, Tang Z, Gao S, Li C, Feng Y, Zhou X. Tumor-associated macrophages: Recent insights and therapies. Frontiers in Oncology. 2020;**10**:188. DOI: 10.3389/fonc.2020.00188

[44] Crezee T, Rabold K, de Jong L, Jaeger M, Netea-Maier R. Metabolic programming of tumor associated macrophages in the context of cancer treatment. Annals of Translational Medicine. 2020;**8**(16):1028. DOI: 10.21037/atm-20-1114

[45] Zhang Q, Wang J, Yadav DK, Bai X, Liang T. Glucose metabolism: The metabolic signature of tumor associated

macrophage. Frontiers in Immunology. 2021;**12**:702580. DOI: 10.3389/fimmu.2021.702580

[46] Liu Y, Xu R, Gu H, et al. Metabolic reprogramming in macrophage responses. Biomarker Research. 2021;**9**:1. DOI: 10.1186/s40364-020-00251-y

[47] Zhu X, Guo Y, Liu Z, Yang J, Tang H, Wang Y. Itaconic acid exerts anti-inflammatory and antibacterial effects via promoting pentose phosphate pathway to produce ROS. Scientific Reports. 2021;**11**(1):18173. DOI: 10.1038/s41598-021-97352-x

[48] Szondi DC, Wong JK, Vardy LA, Cruickshank SM. Arginase signalling as a key player in chronic wound pathophysiology and healing. Frontiers in Molecular Biosciences. 2021;**8**:773866. DOI: 10.3389/fmolb.2021.773866

[49] Viola A, Munari F, Sánchez-Rodríguez R, Scolaro T, Castegna A. The metabolic signature of macrophage responses. Frontiers in Immunology. 2019;**10**:1462. DOI: 10.3389/fimmu.2019.01462

[50] Boutilier AJ, Elsawa SF. Macrophage polarization states in the tumor microenvironment. International Journal of Molecular Sciences. 2021;**22**(13):6995. DOI: 10.3390/ijms22136995

[51] Yao Y, Xu X, Jin L. Macrophage polarization in physiological and pathological pregnancy. Frontiers in Immunology. 2018. DOI: 10.3389/fimmu.2019.00792

[52] Mantovani A, Marchesi F, Malesci A, Laghi L, Allavena P. Tumour-associated macrophages as treatment targets in oncology. Nature Reviews. Clinical Oncology. 2017;**14**(7):399-416. DOI: 10.1038/nrclinonc.2016.217

[53] Komohara Y, Fujiwara Y, Ohnishi K, Takeya M. Tumor-associated macrophages: Potential therapeutic targets for anti-cancer therapy. Advanced Drug Delivery Reviews. 2016;**99**(Pt B):180-185. DOI: 10.1016/j.addr.2015.11.009

Section 3

Cell Interactions and Signaling in Cancer

Chapter 6

Perspective Chapter: Critical Role of Hedgehog in Tumor Microenvironment

Xing-Guo Li and Jer-Yen Yang

Abstract

Hedgehog (Hh) signaling is a highly conserved pathway that plays a pivotal role during embryonic development. Mounting evidence has implicated Hh signaling in various types of cancer. Accordingly, inhibition of aberrant Hh signaling continues to be pursed across multiple cancer types -with some success in certain malignancies. In addition, with the renaissance of antitumor immunotherapy, an in-depth understanding of the molecular mechanisms underlying how the multifaceted functions of Hh signaling shape immunologically suppressive tumor microenvironment might be the key to unlocking a new era of oncological treatments associated with a reduced propensity for the development of drug resistance. Here, we focus on the latest advances regarding the immunological effects of misregulation of Hh signaling on tumor immunity. We also review the current status of clinically approved Hh inhibitors and dissect the mechanisms of drug resistance. Finally, we discuss the potential clinical applications that harness the immunomodulatory effects of Hh signaling not only to circumvent drug resistance, but also to achieve durable efficacy following immunotherapies, thus ultimately resulting in improved patient outcomes.

Keywords: hedgehog signaling, tumor microenvironment, immune cell, smoothened inhibitors, therapeutic targeting

1. Introduction

The Hedgehog (Hh) signaling pathway was discovered as a key regulator of organ development in *Drosophila melanogaster* by Christiane Nüsslein-Vollhard and Eric Wieschaus in the 1980s [1]. It was named after the gene locus associated with a spiky appearance of "hedgehog" phenotype in mutant *Drosophila* larve, findings based on which both investigators were awarded the Nobel Prize in Physiology or Medicine in 1995 "for their discoveries concerning the genetic control of early embryonic development," together with Edward B. Lewis [2]. Since then, the Hh signaling has been extensively studied as a highly conserved evolutionary pathway to orchestrate embryonic development, cell growth and differentiation, homeostasis [3]. Unlike other classical signaling cascades, Hh signaling is almost silent in the adult organisms but reactivated in a few tissues such as the skin, during tissue regeneration and wound

IntechOpen

healing [3]. Not surprisingly, aberrant activation of this pathway has been demonstrated as a potent oncogenic driver to promote numerous hallmarks of cancer [4]. Therefore, the multifaceted role of Hh signaling may allow exploitation of this key pathway for novel and more effective cancer therapy [5].

Activation of Hh signaling is dependent on the primary cilium, a highly specialized organelle found on most vertebrate cells. Three Hh ligands, sonic hedgehog (Shh), desert hedgehog (Dhh), and Indian hedgehog (Ihh), are known to actuate the Hh pathway during embryonic and tissue development [6]. Whereas the expression patterns for Dhh and Ihh are tissue-specific, Shh has a broader expression pattern in various compartments and in multiple developmental stages [6]. In general, the Hh signaling is activated through either canonical or non-canonical mechanisms. In the canonical pathway, Hh ligands bind to the surface receptor Patched 1 (PTCH1), which alleviates the inhibitory effect of PTCH1 on a G-protein-coupled receptor (GPCR)-like protein, Smoothened (SMO), leading to migration of SMO to the tip of the cilium, which in turn signals suppressor of fused (SUFU) to release glioma-associated oncogene homolog proteins (GLIs). Finally, GLIs translocate into the nucleus, resulting in a signaling cascade through transcriptional regulation of Hh target genes [6]. Alternatively, GLI transcription factors can be activated through non-canonical mechanisms, which can be independently of PTCH1, SMO, or both [6]. Of note, mounting evidence has demonstrated that the signaling pathways that can induce non-canonical Hh signaling have been of known significance in oncogenesis, providing the mechanistic basis of the cross talk between Hh signaling and other signaling pathways to promote tumorigenesis, as well as the rationale for development of potential combination therapeutics [7–10].

The discovery of PTCH mutations in basal cell nevus syndrome (BCNS, or Gorlin syndrome, or nevoid basal cell carcinoma [BCC] syndrome), a hereditary form of BCC, provides the first link between the Hh signaling and tumorigenesis [11, 12]. Other than BCC, emerging evidence has involved abnormal activation of Hh signaling in a variety of cancer types, such as medulloblastoma, breast cancer, pancreatic cancer, and lung cancer [13].

So far, three models have been proposed to elucidate the role of Hh signaling in oncogenesis where Hh signaling is over-activated through ligand production, autocrine, juxtacrine, or paracrine reception of the ligand, as well as cross talk between Hh signaling and complex intracellular signaling cascades [13]. First, in BCC and medulloblastoma, activating mutations of Hh pathway have been identified, such as inactivating mutations in PTCH or SUFU, and activating mutations in SMO, as shown in 85% of sporadic BCC or 30% of medulloblastoma, respectively [11–16]. In this scenario, the autonomous activation of Hh signaling is independent of Hh ligands.

Second, Hh signaling is aberrantly activated through autocrine or juxtacrine ligand-dependent manner, where Hh is secreted and responded by the same or adjacent cells [13]. This category of cancers includes breast cancer, pancreatic cancer, lung cancer, prostate cancer, colorectal cancer, stomach and esophageal cancer, ovarian and endometrial cancer, melanomas, and gliomas [13]. Finally, in pancreatic cancer, prostate cancer, and colon cancer, Hh signaling is activated through a paracrine-dependent manner, where Hh ligands are secreted by tumor cells, whereas the PTCH receptor is expressed on stromal cells in the tumor microenvironment (TME). In this last model of Hh signaling activation, a feedback loop is generated, which allows the transmit of the growth-promoting signals from tumor cells to stromal cells and then back to tumor cells, leading to sustained tumor progression [17].

In the following sections, we will first highlight the key cellular components of TME involved in oncogenic Hh signaling to promote tumor progression. We will then review the current status of the FDA-approved and non-approved inhibitors of Hh signaling, as well as the molecular mechanisms of drug resistance. Finally, we will provide a critical evaluation of recent studies on the treatments combining immunotherapeutic strategies with approved Hh inhibitors and will propose potential strategies that could be applied to harness existing knowledge to overcome the drug resistance.

2. The role of Hh signaling in the TME

Emerging evidence has suggested that TME is not just a silent bystander, but rather an active player of tumor progression [18, 19]. The composition of TME not only varies between tumor types, but also is continuously evolving in the different stages of tumorigenesis. Hh signaling has been intensively studied with respect to the classical hallmarks of cancer [3–6]. In contrast, its role in the modulation of TME has only become evident in recent studies [20–22].

2.1 Immune cells

The adaptive and innate immune systems cooperate to form a highly proficient immune surveillance machinery that can identify and eradicate genetically altered cells to prevent tumorigenesis. Tumor-infiltrating leukocytes (TILs), including T and B lymphocytes, monocytes and macrophages, myeloid-derived suppressor cells (MDSCs), dendritic cells (DCs), and natural killer (NK) cells, play diverse roles in tumor progression through interactions and production of cytokines, chemokines, and growth factors to support or suppress tumor growth and metastasis [20, 21]. There is increasing evidence from multiple experimental models that demonstrate an important and multifaceted role of Hh signaling in the modulation of immune cell functions. Aberrant Hh signaling induces a hostile, immunosuppressive microenvironment to dampen an effective antitumor immune response.

Regulatory T cells (Tregs) control the activity of effector immune cells such as granzyme B-expressing $CD8^+$ T cells and NK cells by secreting anti-inflammatory cytokines such as TGF-β and interleukin-10 (IL-10) [23]. The immune modulatory role of Hh signaling in T cells is evidenced by recent studies demonstrating that Hh signaling may directly regulate the expression and activity of TGF-β. Treg infiltration has been described for Hh-associated tumors, such as BCC [24], and medulloblastoma [25–28].

Intriguingly, elevated Treg infiltration is accompanied by an increase of TGF-β within intra- and peri-tumoral skin in a human UV-exposed facial BCC model [29]. In line with the putative immunosuppressive phenotype of Hh signaling, genetic abrogation of T-cell TGF-β signaling mitigated tumor progression in a transgenic medulloblastoma mouse model overexpressing smoothened A1 (SmoA1), an obligatory and conserved Hh signal transducer [25]. In this study, TGF-β signaling blockade led to nearly abolishment of Tregs and licensing of CD8 cytotoxic T lymphocytes for antitumor immunity [23].

Mechanistically, GLI2, an Hh effector, has been shown to directly activate the expression of TGF-β in human Tregs [30]. Thus, it has been proposed that Hh signaling may help generate a feed-forward loop where TGF-β induces the inversion of $CD4^+$ T cells to Tregs, which in turn secrete high levels of TGF-β, leading to enforcement of the continued presence of immunosuppressive Tregs in the tumor microenvironment [31].

Myeloid cell infiltration has been described in multiple cancer entities where tumors may benefit from myeloid cells-mediated immunosuppression. The role of Hh signaling in the tumor-promoting function of myeloid cells has been postulated based on observations in multiple models of Hh-induced tumors. First, in a murine SMO-induced BCC model, tumor growth appears to be enhanced by the recruitment of immunosuppressive myeloid derived suppressor cells (MDSCs), accompanied by a reduction of effector lymphocytes in the tumor lesions [32]. This is mediated by the TGF-β-CCL2 (C-C motif chemokine ligand 2) axis secreted by oncogenic SMO-expressing keratinocytes and the CCL2 receptor expressed by MDSCs. *In vivo*, pharmacological suppression of the CCL2 receptor expression decreased infiltration of MDSCs and resulted in reduced tumor growth, indicating an immunosuppressive phenotype by the oncogenic Hh signaling [33]. Likewise, there is also strong evidence for immunosuppressive function of myeloid cells in Hh-associated medulloblastomas, which are characterized by high myeloid infiltration. For example, gene expression profiling of human Hh medulloblastoma tumors showed enrichment for an M2-like gene expression profile, consistent with immunosuppressive functions of myeloid cells [34]. Moreover, an inverse correlation has been observed between expression of M2-like markers (such as CD163) and survival of human Hh medulloblastoma patients [34].

Along these lines, the notion of an immunosuppressive function of Hh signaling was further affirmed by two recent studies in Hh-induced medulloblastomas. In a mouse model of Hh medulloblastoma ($Ptch1^{+/-}$; $Tp53^{-/-}$), Dang et al. showed decreased T-cell proliferation in a co-culture system of tumor-infiltrating myeloid cells and *ex vivo* stimulated T cells [35]. Mechanistically, the immunosuppressive phenotype appears to be mediated by CCL2. Genetic knockout of CCL2 receptor not only decreased infiltration of monocyte-derived macrophages but also increased levels of $CD8^+$ T cells in tumors [35]. Likewise, in another mouse model of Hh-induced medulloblastoma (Atoh1-SmoM2), pharmacological inhibition of colony stimulating factor 1 receptor (CSF1R) depleted macrophages and microglia, resulting in delayed tumor growth and prolonged mouse survival [36]. These recent studies support the notion of a tumor- promoting function of macrophages, which are consistent with an early study in another Hh-associated medulloblastoma tumor model, where the presence of MDSCs increases infiltration of Tregs and reduces the number of effector T cells [37]. Interestingly, infiltrating myeloid cells have been described as the predominant source of PD-L1 expression in a mouse model of Hh-induced medulloblastoma where the binding of PD- L1 to PD-1 on effector T cells resulted in T-cell exhaustion and immune escape of tumor cells [38]. Furthermore, an analysis of an immunocompetent breast cancer xenograft mouse model showed that inhibition of Hh signaling (SMO inhibitor vismodegib) led to reduced infiltration of immunosuppressive myeloid cells in the tumors, accompanied by an increase of effector $CD8^+$ T cells and M1 macrophages [39].

2.2 Tumor-associated astrocytes (TAAs)

Astrocytes, the most abundant type of glial cells in the brain, are integral partners with neurons in the regulation of neuronal development and brain function. Hh signaling has emerged as a critical player to support astrocyte-mediated modulation of neuronal activity [40–42]. A recent series of elegant work supports a key role of tumor-associated astrocytes (TAAs) in promoting tumor growth and metastasis through distinct signaling, including Hh pathway [43–46]. First, TAAs were shown to secret the ligand Shh, which is required for maintaining cell proliferation of Hh-activated medulloblastoma through a Smo-dependent, but Gli1-independent manner, despite the absence of its primary receptor Ptch1. Of note, ablation of TAAs blocked tumor growth [43]. Furthermore, a recent study at single-cell resolution demonstrated that Hh-induced medulloblastoma cells can transdifferentiate into interleukin-4 (IL-4)-secreting TAAs, which in turn stimulates tumor-associated microglia to release insulin-like growth factor 1 (IGF1) to promote tumor progression [44]. Similarly, medulloblastoma-associated astrocytes have recently been shown to produce high levels of CCL2, a tumor-promoting cytokine shown to drive stemness maintenance and proliferation of disseminated tumor cells [45] and to promote metastasis [47]. Moreover, using single-cell RNA sequencing and lineage tracing analyses, Guo et al. investigated cellular origin of TAAs in a mouse model for relapsed Hh-activated medulloblastoma driven by *Ptch1* knockout [46]. This study has elegantly demonstrated that TAAs are predominantly derived from the transdifferentiation of tumor cells in relapsed MB, but not in primary MB, thus establishing the distinct cellular sources of astrocytes [46]. Interestingly, this study revealed that such transdifferentiation of medulloblastoma cells to TAAs depends on bone morphogenetic proteins (BMPs) and that pharmacological inhibition of BMP signaling repressed transdifferentiation and suppressed tumor relapse [46]. It remains to be determined what drives these transdifferentiation events and what intrinsic and extrinsic mechanisms, beyond Hh and BMP signaling, regulate the potential cooperation of TAAs and microglia in promoting the immunosuppressed state of medulloblastoma.

2.3 Cancer-associated fibroblasts (CAFs)

Cancer-associated fibroblasts (CAFs), the most abundant stromal cells in TME, have emerged as a central player in cancer progression and metastasis [48]. Through diverse phenotypes, origins, and functions, CAFs modulate the cross talk between inflammation and tumorigenesis and contribute to therapeutic resistance by producing various cytokines, chemokines, growth factors, and matrix-degrading enzymes [49].

There is increasing evidence indicating that CAF populations that support or suppress tumor growth and progression through stroma-specific Hh activation have been detected in multiple tumor types, including pancreatic cancer, colon cancer, and bladder cancer [50]. Recent advances in single-cell technologies have enabled detailed characterization of the heterogeneity and plasticity of differential CAF subsets, supporting a new therapeutic strategy in which tumor-supporting CAFs are reprogrammed into tumor-suppressing CAFs [50]. In pancreatic ductal adenocarcinoma (PDAC), Hh signaling pathway is activated in CAFs via a paracrine mechanism and has been associated with pancreatic tumorigenesis [49]. Initial studies indicated that inhibition of Hh pathway impaired tumor growth and sensitized tumors to chemotherapy in multiple PDAC models [51–56]. However, recent studies have challenged the concept of tumor-promoting CAFs. In the context of an oncogenic Kras-driven mouse PDAC model, conditional deletion of *Shh*, the predominant Hh ligand expressed in pancreas, led to cachexia and to poorly differentiated and highly vascularized tumors [57].

Moreover, by using three distinctly genetically engineered mouse PDAC models, another study showed that pharmacologic inhibition of Hh pathway activity accelerated rather than delayed progression of oncogenic Kras-driven disease by affecting the balance between epithelial and stroma elements, leading to suppression of stromal desmoplasia but accelerated growth of pancreatic intraepithelial neoplasia [58]. These contradictory findings indicate that Hh signaling may play pleiotropic roles in PDAC progression. Interestingly, by using a combination of pharmacologic inhibition, gain- and loss-of-function genetic experiments, cytometry by time-of-flight, and single-cell RNA sequencing, a more recent study defines dosage-dependent effects of Hh signaling on the composition and function of CAFs in PDAC microenvironment [59]. Hh signaling is uniquely activated and differentially elevated in CAFs, with higher levels in myofibroblastic CAFs (myCAF) compared with inflammatory CAFs (iCAF) in both mouse and human PDAC. Driving high levels of Hh signaling promotes tumor growth, whereas Hh pathway inhibition alters the ratio of myCAF/iCAF populations, which is accompanied by a decrease in cytotoxic T cells and an expansion in regulatory T cells, thus altering the composition of CAFs, and shifting the inflammatory response toward a more immunosuppressive phenotype [59]. Given the differential functional implications for CAF subpopulations, changes in the ratio of CAF subtypes may lead to distinct antitumor outcomes. Consistent with, recent studies demonstrated a possible negative impact of current Hh pathway inhibitors on antitumor response in clinical trials, which were largely unsuccessful or even detrimental to patient health [60, 61]. Further understanding of the roles of Hh signaling in CAFs may open the possibility for more effective combination cancer therapies.

3. Therapeutic targeting Hh signaling in cancers

Given the multifaceted role of Hh signaling in cancer, inhibitors of Hh pathways have emerged as an important class of anticancer agents. These compounds fall into three main categories: Hh ligand inhibitors, SMO inhibitors, and GLI inhibitors [62]. Despite extensive efforts devoted to the discovery of Hh signaling inhibitors, so far only three drugs have been approved by the Food and Drug Administration (FDA), all targeting the upstream receptor of Hh signaling SMO, a membrane protein of the GPCR protein family [62].

3.1 FDA-approved inhibitors

To date, three SMO inhibitors, vismodegib, sonidegib, and glasdegib, have been FDA approved in 2012, 2015, and 2018, respectively, for cancer treatment. Cyclopamine, the first SMO antagonist, is a naturally occurring alkaloid found in the corn lily [63] later proved to bind to SMO and to inhibit activation of downstream Hh target genes [64].

Extensive efforts have been made to develop alkaloid derivatives to increase the bioavailability, sensitivity, and specificity of cyclopamine to target SMO [65]. Vismodegib (GDC-0449 or Erivedge), the first cyclopamine derivative and Hh pathway–targeting drug, is currently approved for the treatment of patients with locally advanced or metastatic BCC (US FDA). Compared to cyclopamine, vismodegib shows a higher potency and more favorable pharmacological properties [62]. The approval of vismodegib was based on results from the pivotal phase II ERIVANCE trial (Clinica lTrials.gov, NCT00833417) showing that vismodegib substantially shrank tumors or healed visible lesions (objective response rate, ORR) in 43% of patients with locally advanced BCC and 30% of patients with metastatic BCC, at 21 months, with a median progression-free survival (PFS) duration of 9.5 months for both metastatic and locally advanced BCC patients [66, 67]. Up to the completion of this manuscript, there have been 86 clinical trials for vismodegib, both monotherapy and combination, in various cancer types (ClinicalTrials.gov).

Sonidegib (Erismodegib, NVP-LDE-225, LDE-225, Odomzo) is another cyclopamine-derived SMO antagonist discovered in 2010 through an *in vitro*, high-throughput screen, showing high tissue penetration and bioavailability, as well as the ability to cross the blood-brain barrier [68]. In 2015, sonidegib became the second SMO inhibitor approved for patients with locally advanced or recurrent BCC (US FDA). The approval of sonidegib was based on results from a multicenter, randomized, double-blind phase II BOLT trial (ClinicalTrials.gov, number NCT01327053), which showed the objective response rates of 38% and 43% in the 800 and 200 mg dosage groups, respectively after 30 months in patients with locally advanced BCC and the objective response rates of 17% and 15%, respectively in those with metastatic BCC [69]. Up to August 2022, there are 46 clinical trials for sonidegib in cancer treatment (ClinicalTrials.gov).

A third FDA-approved inhibitor of Hh signaling is glasdegib (PF-04449913, Daurismo), a benzamide derivative discovered in 2012 with high potency and oral bioavailability [70]. In 2018, glasdegib was approved for combination treatment with low-dose cytarabine arabinoside (LDAC) for patients with acute myeloid leukemia unsuitable for intensive chemotherapy. The approval of glasdegib was based on the results of the phase II BRIGHT 1003 trial (ClinicalTrials.gov, NCT01546038) showing the median overall survival of 8.8 months with glasdegib/LDAC as compared to 4.9 months with LDAC. Furthermore, 17.0% and 2.3% of patients in the glasdegib/LDAC and LDAC arms, respectively, achieved complete remission [71]. Up to this point, there have been 26 clinical trials for glasdegib in various cancer types (Clinica lTrials.gov).

3.2 Resistance mechanisms to FDA-approved inhibitors

The first retrospective study on drug resistance to SMO inhibitor therapy was reported in 2012 where 21% of BCC patients treated with vismodegib developed drug resistance, with a mean tumor recurrence time of 56.4 weeks in clinical examination [72]. Ever since, resistance to SMO antagonists has been observed in patients who never respond to SMO inhibitor therapy (primary resistance), as well as in those who initially respond but later develop resistance to SMO inhibitors (acquired resistance) [73]. Mechanistically, a number of models have been proposed to explain the basis of drug resistance to SMO inhibitor therapy. First, genetic analysis of resistant tumors has revealed mutations of SMO, loss of SUFU, and amplification of GLIs or Hh target genes, such as CCND1 and GLI1 [5, 10]. Second, accumulating evidence supports the notion that the resistance can be driven through the non-canonical Hh signaling, accompanied by the concurrent activation of other oncogenic signaling pathways, such as AP-1 and TGF-β signaling [74], RhoA signaling [75], and RAS-MAPK signaling [76]. Finally, a new mechanism has recently been uncovered to contribute to drug resistance through loss of primary cilia [77, 78]. This was supported by both preclinical and clinical evidence. In Hh-dependent medulloblastoma, recurrent mutations in oral facial digital syndrome 1 (OFD1), a culprit gene led to loss of cilia, and thereby caused resistance to SMO inhibitors [78]. Importantly, sequencing data analysis from resistant BCC patients showed recurrent mutations in ciliary genes, providing clinical relevance of this new mechanism [77]. Therefore, a better understanding of cilia-regulating signaling pathways in resistant cancer may open up a new route to reintroduce cilia to sensitize resistant cancer cells to SMO inhibitors. Taken together, several strategies have been proposed to overcome the drug resistance through targeting the underlying mechanisms. These approaches include: (1) develop second-generation SMO inhibitors to retain anticancer activities that are not affected by the resistance-inducing mutations [5]; (2) target downstream components of SMO, such as GLIs (see below, non- approved inhibitors), or signaling molecules involved in the non-canonical Hh signaling pathway [8].

3.3 Non-FDA-approved inhibitors

Multiple novel inhibitors targeting SMO have been shown to be effective in preclinical models [5] and are now in active clinical trials, either monotherapy or combination for various cancer types. These compounds include saridegib (patidegib, IPI-926), taladegib (LY2940680), and BMS-833923 (XL139) (ClinicalTrials.gov). On the other hand, even though GLI1 antagonists are not as extensive as those targeting SMO, mounting evidence has shown that targeting the Hh signaling at the level of its final effector, GLI1, is a promising strategy to overcome resistance to currently available SMO inhibitors [79, 80]. In this regard, the promising pharmacological potential of direct and indirect GLI inhibitors, as well as GLI antagonists derived from natural products, has been in active investigation at the preclinical or clinical phase. It is anticipated that future study on these compounds will help develop new strategies tackling resistant mechanisms and tumor heterogeneity [81].

4. Hh signaling and antitumor immune response

In 2018, James P Allison and Tasuku Honjo were awarded the Nobel Prize in Physiology or Medicine "for their discovery of cancer therapy by inhibition of negative immune regulation" [82]. Although this breakthrough in cancer immunotherapy has revolutionized cancer treatment, only a subset of patients elicit favorable responses and most immunologically cold solid tumors are not responsive [83]. Given the immunosuppressive function of Hh signaling, inhibitors of Hh signaling pathway may hold promise in converting nonresponsive cold tumors into responsive hot ones, which may subsequently allow nonresponders to benefit from immunotherapies. Notably, clinically approved Hh inhibitors, as well as non-approved inhibitors, have been in active preclinical and clinical trials for combined therapies, including immunotherapies.

The first clinical trial with Hh inhibitors in combination with immune checkpoint inhibitors was conducted in 16 patients with advanced BCC (clincialtrial.gov, NCT02690948). This trial showed that pembrolizumab (PD-L1 inhibitor) is active against BCCs. Although the two groups of pembrolizumab with or without vismodegib were not directly compared, the response rate for the combination group was not superior to the monotherapy group [84]. Of note, most patients with advanced BCC progress on or are intolerant to Hh inhibitor therapy despite objective response rates of 30–60% [66–69, 85]. Until Feb 9, 2021, when cemiplimab, a PD-1 antibody, was approved by the US FDA fully for patients with locally advanced BCC, and accelerated for patients with metastatic BCC, after treatment with Hh inhibitors, or for whom Hh inhibitors are not appropriate [86], there was no standard second-line treatment option for these BCC patients [72]. A recent clinical trial study provides the first report to show clinically meaningful antitumor activity of cemiplimab in patients with BCC after Hh inhibitor therapy ([87], clinicaltrials.gov, NTC03132636). In this trial, the efficacy and safety of cemiplimab were evaluated in patients with locally advanced BCC or metastatic BCC who had previously been treated with an Hh inhibitor. Among the efficacy population (n = 121), centrally reviewed objective response was observed in 31% of patients with estimated duration of response exceeding 1 year in 85% of responders [87].

Importantly, this study also showed that the safety profile was consistent with what is known for immune checkpoint class of drugs, even considering the advanced age of the patient population in the present study [87]. These findings demonstrate the efficacy of immune checkpoint blockade in treating BCC in patients who had previously received Hh inhibitor therapy, thus opening a new horizon for treatment of the many patients who discontinue Hh inhibitor therapy due to disease progression, toxicity, or drug resistance. Moreover, a recent case report demonstrated an impressive response to cemiplimab in a sonidegib-resistant giant basosquamous carcinoma, one form of BCC [88]. Finally, a dozen of clinical trials have been initiated to investigate the combination treatment of anti-PD-1, PD-L1, and CTLA-4 monoclonal antibody therapy with first-line Hh inhibitors in patients with a variety of cancer types (see **Table 1**). The outcome of these trials will not only inform about whether combinatorial treatments can increase the efficacy and duration of antitumor response, but also provide insights into the optimal customized regimen to circumvent resistance to Hh inhibitors.

Comparatively a few recent studies have indicated possible negative effects of the current Hh inhibitor therapy on antitumor immunity [89]. For instance, blockade of SMO signaling may inhibit formation of the immunological synapse [90]. Administration of SMO inhibitors caused the functional disruption of the immunological synapse, leading to the loss of T-cell effector activity [90]. Even though it remains unclear whether Hh inhibitor therapy may impede cytotoxic T-cell killing in cancer patients, a pilot clinical trial study of vismodegib in combination with pembrolizumab did not suggest additive clinical activity [84]. In the clinical context, there is an emerging paradigm that immunotherapy may show the greatest activity when administered early in the natural history of cancers. Further studies are warranted to evaluate the efficacy and duration of immune checkpoint blockade before Hh inhibitor therapy.

5. Conclusions

The Hh signaling pathway has attracted extensive research attention as a key player to contribute to the progression of a variety of human cancer types. With an in-depth understanding of the molecular mechanisms underlying the role of Hh signaling in tumorigenesis, enormous efforts have been made to develop specific inhibitors targeting molecular components of this pathway. Consequently, cancer therapy has undergone a paradigm shift from eradicating tumor cells to multidimensional targeting and normalizing tumor cells and TME. Herein, we reviewed the multifaceted function of Hh signaling in shaping immunologically suppressive TME to promote tumor progression, provided an up-to-date status of active clinical trials of FDA approved Hh inhibitors, and finally, highlighted possible therapeutic interventions that harness the immunomodulatory effects of Hh signaling not only to overcome drug resistance, but also to achieve durable efficacy following immunotherapies.

SMO inhibitor	Combination	Cancer Type	Enrollment	Phase	Status	NCT #
Vismodegib (GDC-0449 or Erivedge)	+ VEGF-A antibody and chemotherapy	Metastatic Colorectal Cancer	199	Phase 2	Completed	NCT00636610
	+ Anti-hormone therapy	Prostate Cancer	10	Phase 1|2	Terminated	NCT01163084
	+ Chemotherapy	Pancreatic Cancer	118	Phase 1|2	Completed	NCT01064622
	+ VEGF-A antibody and chemotherapy	Ovarian Cancer|Basal Cell Carcinoma|Metastatic Colorectal Cancer	19	Phase 2	Completed	NCT00959647
	+ Notch inhibitor	Breast Cancer	13	Phase 1	Terminated	NCT01071564
	+ Chemotherapy	Gastric Cancer	124	Phase 2	Completed	NCT00982592
	+ Chemotherapy	Pancreatic Cancer	25	Phase 2	Completed	NCT01195415
	+ Chemotherapy	Myelodysplastic Syndromes,	38	Phase 2	Terminated	NCT01880437
	+ Notch inhibitor	Sarcoma	78 Phase1|2	Completed	NCT01154452	
	+ Photodynamic therapy	Basal Cell Nevus Syndrome	24	Phase 2	Completed	NCT01556009
	+ IGF1R antibody and chemotherapy	Small Cell Lung Carcinoma	168	Phase 2	Completed	NCT00887159
	+ Chemotherapy	Pancreatic Adenocarcinoma	21	Phase 1	Unknown	NCT01713218
	+ Chemotherapy	Medulloblastoma	24	Phase 1|2	Terminated	NCT01601184
	+ Chemotherapy	Metastatic Pancreatic Cancer	98	Phase 2	Completed	NCT01088815
	+ DNMT inhibitor	Acute Myeloid Leukemia	40	Phase 2	Unknown	NCT02073838
	+ mTOR inhibitor	Pancreatic Cancer	31	Phase 1	Completed	NCT01537107
	+ PD1 blockade	Skin Basal Cell Carcinoma	16	Phase 1|2	Completed	NCT02690948
	+ Chemotherapy	Breast Cancer	40	Phase 2	Unknown	NCT02694224
	+ Radiation therapy	Basal Cell Carcinoma	24	Phase 2	Completed	NCT01835626
	+ Radiation therapy	Carcinoma, Basal Cell	14	Phase 2	Terminated	NCT02956889

DOI: http://dx.doi.org/10.5772/intechopen.108831

SMO inhibitor	Combination	Cancer Type	Enrollment	Phase	Status	NCT #
	+ PD1/CTLA4 blockade	Basal Cell Nevus Syndrome	0	Phase 2	Withdrawn	NCT03767439
	+ Tyrosine kinase inhibitor	Basal Cell Carcinoma	84	Phase 2	Recruiting	NCT04416516
	+ Tyrosine kinase inhibitors and PARP inhibitors	Miscellaneous	950	Phase 2	Recruiting	NCT02925234
	+ PDL1 blockade and Tyrosine kinase inhibitors	Miscellaneous	676	Phase 2	Active, not recruiting	NCT02091141
	+ PDL1 blockade, Tyrosine kinase inhibitors and chemotherapy	Lymphoma, Non-Hodgkin	720	Phase 2	Recruiting	NCT03297606
	+ PDL1 blockade, Tyrosine kinase inhibitors and chemotherapy	Cancer of Unknown Primary Site	790	Phase 2	Recruiting	NCT03498521
	+ PDL1 blockade, Tyrosine kinase inhibitors and chemotherapy	Miscellaneous	384	Phase 2	Recruiting	NCT04591431
	+ Targeted therapy and chemotherapy	Glioblastoma, Adult	350	Phase 1|2	Recruiting	NCT03158389
	+ Targeted therapy and chemotherapy	Meningioma	124	Phase 2	Recruiting	NCT02523014
	+ PDL1 blockade, Tyrosine kinase inhibitors and chemotherapy	Miscellaneous	300	Phase 2	Recruiting	NCT04341181
	+ PDL1 blockade, Tyrosine kinase inhibitors and chemotherapy	Miscellaneous	6452	Phase 2	Recruiting	NCT02465060
	+ PDL1 blockade, Tyrosine kinase inhibitors and chemotherapy	Miscellaneous 40	Phase 1	Recruiting	NCT03878524	
	+ PDL1 blockade, Tyrosine kinase inhibitors and chemotherapy	Miscellaneous	131	Phase 2	Not yet recruiting	NCT05238831
	+ PDL1 blockade, Tyrosine kinase inhibitors and chemotherapy	Advanced Cancer|Solid Tumor	250	Phase 2	Recruiting	NCT05159245

SMO inhibitor	Combination	Cancer Type	Enrollment	Phase	Status	NCT #
	+ Radiation therapy and chemotherapy	Medulloblastoma	660	Phase 2	Recruiting	NCT01878617
	+ PDL1 blockade	Cancer Metastatic	1000	Phase 2	Recruiting	NCT04817956
	+ Chemotherapy	Pancreatic Cancer	55	Phase 1	Active, not recruiting	NCT00878163
Sonidegib (Erismodegib, NVP-LDE-225, LDE-225, Odomzo)	+ Radiation therapy and chemotherapy	Medulloblastoma	205	Phase 2	Not yet recruiting NCT04402073	
	+ Chemotherapy	Lung Cancer	19	Phase 1	Completed	NCT01579929
	+ JAK inhibitor	Miscellaneous	50	Phase 1|2	Completed	NCT01787552
	+ Chemotherapy	Pancreatic Ductal Adenocarcinoma	23	Phase 1|2	Terminated	NCT01431794
	+ Chemotherapy	Myelodysplastic Syndrome	63	Phase 1	Completed	NCT02129101
	+ mTOR kinase inhibitor	Esophageal Cancer	25	Phase 1	Completed	NCT02138929
	+ Chemotherapy	Plasma Cell Myeloma	28	Phase 2	Completed	NCT02086552
	+ Chemotherapy	Pancreatic Cancer	78	Phase 1|2	Completed	NCT02358161
	+ Tyrosine kinase inhibitor and chemotherapy	Chronic Myelogenous Leukemia	11	Phase 1	Completed	NCT01456676
	+ Tyrosine kinase inhibitor and chemotherapy	Miscellaneous	108	Phase 1	Recruiting	NCT03434262
	+ Tyrosine kinase inhibitor	Miscellaneous	120	Phase 1	Completed	NCT01576666
	+ Chemotherapy	Advanced Breast Cancer	12	Phase 1	Completed	NCT02027376
	+ Tyrosine kinase inhibitor	Carcinoma, Basal Cell	10	Phase 2	Terminated	NCT02303041
	+ Chemotherapy	Pancreatic Cancer	18	Phase 1	Completed	NCT01487785
	+ PD1 blockade	Miscellaneous	45	Phase 1	Recruiting	NCT04007744
	Neoadjuvant + Surgery	Basal Cell Carcinoma	10	Phase 2	Recruiting	NCT03534947
	+ Chemotherapy	Multiple Myeloma	7	Phase 2	Terminated	NCT02254551

SMO inhibitor	Combination	Cancer Type	Enrollment	Phase	Status	NCT #
	+ Chemotherapy	Solid Tumor|Ovarian Cancer	30	Phase 1	Completed	NCT01954355
	+ Chemotherapy	Pancreatic Cancer	39	Phase 1	Completed	NCT01485744
	+ Chemotherapy	Prostate Cancer	0	Phase 1	Withdrawn	NCT02182622
	+ PD1 blockade	Basal Cell Carcinoma	20	Phase 2	Recruiting	NCT04679480
Glasdegib (PF-04449913, Daurismo)	+ Chemotherapy	Glioblastoma	75	Phase 1|2	Active, not recruiting	NCT03466450
	+ Chemotherapy	Acute Myelogenous Leukemia	30	Phase 2	Recruiting	NCT04231851
	+ Antibody-drug conjugate	Acute Myeloid Leukemia	414	Phase 3	Recruiting	NCT04168502
	+ Chemotherapy	ACUTE MYELOID LEUKEMIA	1	Phase 2	Terminated	NCT04051996
	+ Chemotherapy	Acute Myeloid Leukemia	15	Phase 3	Active, not recruiting	NCT04842604
	+ Chemotherapy	Myelodysplastic Syndrome	73	Phase 1	Completed	NCT02367456
	+ Chemotherapy	Leukemia, Myeloid, Acute	730	Phase 3	Completed	NCT03416179
	+ Chemotherapy	Acute Myeloid Leukemia	0	Phase 1	Withdrawn	NCT04655391
	+ Antibody-drug conjugate	Acute Myeloid Leukemia	28	Phase 3	Terminated	NCT04093505
	+ PD1 blockade, antibody-drug conjugate and chemotherapy	Acute Myeloid Leukemia	138	Phase 1|2	Active, not recruiting	NCT03390296
	+ Chemotherapy	Acute Myeloid Leukemia	48	Phase 1	Active, not recruiting	NCT02038777
	+ Chemotherapy	Leukemia, Myeloid, Acute	0		Withdrawn	NCT04230564
	+ Chemotherapy	Acute Myeloid Leukemia	255	Phase 2	Completed	NCT01546038
	+ Chemotherapy	Adult Acute Myeloid Leukemia	75	Phase 2	Recruiting	NCT03226418
	+ Chemotherapy	Soft Tissue Sarcoma	960	Phase 3	Recruiting	NCT03784014
	+ Chemotherapy and radiation therapy	Glioblastoma	30	Phase 1|2	Not yet recruiting	NCT03529448

SMO inhibitor	Combination	Cancer Type	Enrollment	Phase	Status	NCT #
Saridegib (patidegib, IPI-926)	+ Chemotherapy	Metastatic Pancreatic Cancer	122	Phase 1|2	Completed	NCT01130142
	+ Chemotherapy	Pancreatic Cancer	15	Phase 1	Completed	NCT01383538
	+ Tyrosine kinase inhibitor	Head and Neck Cancer	9	Phase 1	Completed	NCT01255800
Taladegib (LY2940680)	+ Chemotherapy and radiation therapy	Esophageal Adenocarcinoma	7	Phase 1|2	Completed	NCT02530437
	+ Chemotherapy	Small Cell Lung Carcinoma	26	Phase 1|2	Terminated	NCT01722292
	+ Chemotherapy and CDK inhibitors	Breast Cancer|Colon Cancer|Cholangiocarcinoma|Soft Tissue Sarcoma	94	Phase 1	Completed	NCT02784795
BMS-833923 (XL139)	+ Tyrosine kinase inhibitor	Leukemia	33	Phase 1|2	Completed	NCT01218477
	+ Tyrosine kinase inhibitor	Leukemia	70	Phase 2	Terminated	NCT01357655
	+ Chemotherapy	Small Cell Lung Carcinoma	5	Phase 1	Completed	NCT00927875
	+ Chemotherapy	Stomach Neoplasms|Esophageal Neoplasms 39	Phase 1	Completed	NCT00909402	
	+ Proteasome inhibitors	Advanced Cancer, Various, NOS	27	Phase 1	Completed	NCT00884546

Data from clinicaltrials.gov (accessed on 2022/8/22).

Table 1.
Combination therapy of SMO inhibitors under clinical trials.

Acknowledgements

This book chapter was in part of supported by MOST 110-2311-B-039-001, MOST 111-2320-B-039-050 and CMU109-YT-03 (X.-G.L.) and MOST 111-2320-B-039-015 and CMU109-YT-02 (J.-Y.Y.).

Author dctails

Xing-Guo Li[1,2] and Jer-Yen Yang[1,2]*

1 Graduate Institute of Biomedical Science, China Medical University, Taichung, Taiwan

2 Institute of Biochemistry and Molecular Biology, China Medical University, Taichung, Taiwan

*Address all correspondence to: jyyang@cmu.edu.tw

References

[1] Nüsslein-Volhard C, Wieschaus E. Mutations affecting segment number and polarity in drosophila. Nature. 1980; **287**(5785):795-801. DOI: 10.1038/287795a0

[2] The Nobel Prize in Physiology or Medicine. 1995. Available from: https://www.nobelprize.org/prizes/medicine/1995/nusslein-volhard/facts/

[3] Briscoe J, Thérond PP. The mechanisms of hedgehog signalling and its roles in development and disease. Nature Reviews. Molecular Cell Biology. 2013;**14**(7):416-429. DOI: 10.1038/nrm3598

[4] Wu F, Zhang Y, Sun B, McMahon AP, Wang Y. Hedgehog signaling: From basic biology to cancer therapy. Cell Chemical Biology. 2017;**24**(3):252-280. DOI: 10.1016/j.chembiol.2017.02.010

[5] Nguyen NM, Cho J. Hedgehog pathway inhibitors as targeted cancer therapy and strategies to overcome drug resistance. International Journal of Molecular Sciences. 2022;**23**(3):1733. DOI: 10.3390/ijms23031733

[6] Kong JH, Siebold C, Rohatgi R. Biochemical mechanisms of vertebrate hedgehog signaling. Development. 2019; **146**(10):dev166892. DOI: 10.1242/dev.166892

[7] Brechbiel J, Miller-Moslin K, Adjei AA. Crosstalk between hedgehog and other signaling pathways as a basis for combination therapies in cancer. Cancer Treatment Reviews. 2014;**40**(6):750-759. DOI: 10.1016/j.ctrv.2014.02.003

[8] Pietrobono S, Gagliardi S, Stecca B. Non-canonical hedgehog signaling pathway in cancer: Activation of GLI transcription factors beyond smoothened. Frontiers in Genetics. 2019; **10**:556. DOI: 10.3389/fgene.2019.00556

[9] Li YH, Luo J, Mosley YY, Hedrick VE, Paul LN, Chang J, et al. AMP-activated protein kinase directly phosphorylates and destabilizes hedgehog pathway transcription factor GLI1 in Medulloblastoma. Cell Reports. 2015; **12**(4):599-609. DOI: 10.1016/j.celrep.2015.06.054

[10] Gampala S, Zhang G, Chang CJ, Yang JY. Activation of AMPK sensitizes medulloblastoma to Vismodegib and overcomes Vismodegib-resistance. FASEB Bioadvances. 2021;**3**(6):459-469. DOI: 10.1096/fba.2020-00032

[11] Hahn H, Wicking C, Zaphiropoulos PG, Gailani MR, Shanley S, Chidambaram A, et al. Mutations of the human homolog of drosophila patched in the nevoid basal cell carcinoma syndrome. Cell. 1996;**85**:841-851

[12] Johnson RL, Rothman AL, Xie J, Goodrich LV, Bare JW, Bonifas JM, et al. Human homolog of patched, a candidate gene for the basal cell nevus syndrome. Science. 1996;**272**:1668-1671

[13] Amakye D, Jagani Z, Dorsch M. Unraveling the therapeutic potential of the hedgehog pathway in cancer. Nature Medicine. 2013;**19**(11):1410-1422. DOI: 10.1038/nm.3389

[14] Raffel C, Jenkins RB, Frederick L, Hebrink D, Alderete B, Fults DW, et al. Sporadic Medulloblastomas contain PTCH mutations. Cancer Research. 1997; **57**:842-845

[15] Xie J, Murone M, Luoh S-M, Ryan A, Gu Q, Zhang C, et al. Activating smoothened mutations in sporadic basal-cell carcinoma. Nature. 1998;**391**:90-92

[16] Taylor MD, Liu L, Raffel C, Hui C-C, Mainprize TG, Zhang X, et al. Mutations in SUFU predispose to medulloblastoma. Nature Genetics. 2002;**31**:306-310

[17] Theunissen J-W, de Sauvage FJ. Paracrine hedgehog signaling in cancer. Cancer Research. 2009;**69**:6007-6010

[18] Truffi M, Sorrentino L, F. Corsi fibroblasts in the tumor microenvironment. Advances in Experimental Medicine and Biology. 2020;**1234**:15-29

[19] Nicole M, Anderson M, Simon C. The tumor microenvironment. Current Biology. 2020;**30**(16):R921-R925. DOI: 10.1016/j.cub.2020.06.081

[20] Gampala S, Yang JY. Hedgehog pathway inhibitors against tumor microenvironment. Cell. 2021;**10**(11): 3135. DOI: 10.3390/cells10113135

[21] Onishi H, Nakamura K, Yanai K, Nagai S, Nakayama K, Oyama Y, et al. Cancer therapy that targets the hedgehog signaling pathway considering the cancer microenvironment (review). Oncology Reports. 2022;**47**(5):93. DOI: 10.3892/or.2022.8304

[22] Binnewies M, Roberts EW, Kersten K, Chan V, Fearon DF, Merad M, et al. Understanding the tumor immune microenvironment (TIME) for effective therapy. Nature Medicine. 2018;**24**(5):541-550. DOI: 10.1038/s41591-018-0014-x

[23] Shan F, Somasundaram A, Bruno TC, Workman CJ, Vignali DAA. Therapeutic targeting of regulatory T cells in cancer. Trends Cancer. 2022; **S2405-8033**(22):00136-00134. DOI: 10.1016/j.trecan.2022.06.008

[24] O'Donnell JS, Teng MWL, Smyth MJ. Cancer immunoediting and resistance to T cell-based immunotherapy. Nature Reviews. Clinical Oncology. 2019;**16**(3):151-167. DOI: 10.1038/s41571-018-0142-8

[25] Gate D, Danielpour M, Rodriguez J Jr, Kim G-B, Levy R, Bannykh S, et al. T-cell TGF-β signaling abrogation restricts medulloblastoma progression. Proceedings of the National Academy of Sciences. 2014;**111**:E3458-E3466. DOI: 10.1073/pnas.1412489111

[26] Bockmayr M, Mohme M, Klauschen F, Winkler B, Budczies J, Rutkowski S, et al. Subgroup-specific immune and stromal microenvironment in medulloblastoma. Oncoimmunology. 2018;**7**:e1462430. DOI: 10.1080/2162402X.2018.1462430

[27] Vermeulen JF, Van Hecke W, Adriaansen EJM, Jansen MK, Bouma RG, Villacorta Hidalgo J, et al. Prognostic relevance of tumor-infiltrating lymphocytes and immune checkpoints in pediatric medulloblastoma. Oncoimmunology. 2018;**7**:e1398877. DOI: 10.1080/2162402X.2017.1398877

[28] Grabovska Y, Mackay A, O'Hare P, Crosier S, Finetti M, Schwalbe EC, et al. Pediatric pan-central nervous system tumor analysis of immune-cell infiltration identifies correlates of antitumor immunity. Nature Communications. 2020;**11**:4324. DOI: 10.1038/s41467-020-18070-y

[29] Omland SH, Nielsen PS, Gjerdrum LM, Gniadecki R. Immunosuppressive environment in basal cell carcinoma: The role of regulatory T cells. Acta Dermato-Venereologica. 2016;**96**:917-921. DOI: 10.2340/00015555-2440

[30] Furler RL, Uittenbogaart CH. GLI2 regulates TGF-beta1 in human CD4+ T cells: Implications in cancer and HIV

pathogenesis. PLoS One. 2012;**7**:e40874. DOI: 10.1371/journal.pone.0040874

[31] Eisemann T, Wechsler-Reya RJ. Genes & Development. 2022;**36**(9–10): 514-532

[32] Fan Q, Gu D, Liu H, Yang L, Zhang X, Yoder MC, et al. Defective TGF- beta signaling in bone marrow-derived cells prevents hedgehoginduced skin tumors. Cancer Research. 2014;**74**:471-483. DOI: 10.1158/0008-5472.CAN-13-2134-T

[33] Fan Q, He M, Sheng T, Zhang X, Sinha M, Luxon B, et al. Requirement of TGFbeta signaling for SMO-mediated carcinogenesis. The Journal of Biological Chemistry. 2010;**285**:36570-36576. DOI: 10.1074/jbc.C110.164442

[34] Margol AS, Robison NJ, Gnanachandran J, Hung LT, Kennedy RJ, Vali M, et al. Tumor-associated macrophages in SHH subgroup of medulloblastomas. Clinical Cancer Research. 2015;**21**:1457-1465. DOI: 10.1158/1078-0432.CCR-14-1144

[35] Dang MT, Gonzalez MV, Gaonkar KS, Rathi KS, Young P, Arif S, et al. Macrophages in SHH subgroup medulloblastoma display dynamic heterogeneity that varies with treatment modality. Cell Reports. 2021;**34**:108917. DOI: 10.1016/j.celrep.2021.108917

[36] Tan IL, Arifa RDN, Rallapalli H, Kana V, Lao Z, Sanghrajka RM, et al. CSF1R inhibition depletes tumor-associated macrophages and attenuates tumor progression in a mouse sonic hedgehog-Medulloblastoma model. Oncogene. 2021;**40**:396-407. DOI: 10.1038/s41388-020-01536-0

[37] Abad C, Nobuta H, Li J, Kasai A, Yong WH, Waschek JA. Targeted STAT3 disruption in myeloid cells alters immunosuppressor cell abundance in a murine model of spontaneous medulloblastoma. Journal of Leukocyte Biology. 2014;**95**:357-367. DOI: 10.1189/jlb.1012531

[38] Pham CD, Flores C, Yang C, Pinheiro EM, Yearley JH, Sayour EJ, et al. Differential immune microenvironments and response to immune checkpoint blockade among molecular subtypes of murine medulloblastoma. Clinical Cancer Research. 2016;**22**:582-595. DOI: 10.1158/1078-0432.CCR-15-0713

[39] Hanna A, Metge BJ, Bailey SK, Chen D, Chandrashekar DS, Varambally S, et al. Inhibition of hedgehog signaling reprograms the dysfunctional immune microenvironment in breast cancer. Oncoimmunology. 2019;**8**:1548241. DOI: 10.1080/2162402X.2018.1548241

[40] Hill SA, Blaeser AS, Coley AA, Xie Y, Shepard KA, Harwell CC, et al. Sonic hedgehog signaling in astrocytes mediates cell type-specific synaptic organization. eLife. 2019;**8**:e45545. DOI: 10.7554/eLife.45545

[41] Gingrich EC, Case K, Garcia ADR. A subpopulation of astrocyte progenitors defined by sonic hedgehog signaling. Neural Development. 2022;**17**(1):2. DOI: 10.1186/s13064-021-00158-w

[42] Xie Y, Kuan AT, Wang W, Herbert ZT, Mosto O, Olukoya O, et al. Astrocyte-neuron crosstalk through hedgehog signaling mediates cortical synapse development. Cell Reports. 2022;**38**(8):110416. DOI: 10.1016/j.celrep.2022.110416

[43] Liu Y, Yuelling LW, Wang Y, Du F, Gordon RE, O'Brien JA, et al. Astrocytes promote Medulloblastoma progression through hedgehog secretion. Cancer Research. 2017;**77**(23):6692-6703

[44] Yao M, Ventura PB, Jiang Y, Rodriguez FJ, Wang L, Perry JSA, et al. Astrocytic trans-differentiation completes a multicellular paracrine feedback loop required for Medulloblastoma tumor growth. Cell. 2020;**180**(3):502-520.e19

[45] Liu H, Sun Y, O'Brien JA, Franco-Barraza J, Qi X, Yuan H, et al. Necroptotic astrocytes contribute to maintaining stemness of disseminated medulloblastoma through CCL2 secretion. Neuro-Oncology. 2020;**22**: 625-638. DOI: 10.1093/neuonc/noz214

[46] Guo D, Wang Y, Cheng Y, Liao S, Hu J, Du F, et al. Tumor cells generate astrocyte-like cells that contribute to SHH-driven medulloblastoma relapse. The Journal of Experimental Medicine. 2021;**218**(9):e20202350. DOI: 10.1084/jem.20202350

[47] Garzia L, Kijima N, Morrissy AS, De Antonellis P, Guerreiro Stucklin A, Holgado BL, et al. A hematogenous route for medulloblastoma leptomeningeal metastases. Cell. 2018;**172**:1050-1062.e14. DOI: 10.1016/j.cell.2018.01.038

[48] Saw PE, Chen J, Song E. Targeting CAFs to overcome anticancer therapeutic resistance. Trends Cancer. 2022;**8**(7):527-555. DOI: 10.1016/j.trecan.2022.03.001

[49] Lavie D, Ben-Shmuel A, Erez N, Scherz-Shouval R. Cancer-associated fibroblasts in the single-cell era. Nature Cancer. 2022;**3**(7):793-807. DOI: 10.1038/s43018-022-00411-z

[50] Yoshida GJ. Regulation of heterogeneous cancer-associated fibroblasts: The molecular pathology of activated signaling pathways. Journal of Experimental & Clinical Cancer Research. 2020;**39**(1):112. DOI: 10.1186/s13046-020-01611-0

[51] Thayer SP, di Magliano MP, Heiser PW, Nielsen CM, Roberts DJ, Lauwers GY, et al. Hedgehog is an early and late mediator of pancreatic cancer tumorigenesis. Nature. 2003;**425**(6960): 851-856

[52] Berman DM, Karhadkar SS, Maitra A, Montes de Oca R, Gerstenblith MR, Briggs K, et al. Widespread requirement for hedgehog ligand stimulation in growth of digestive tract tumours. Nature. 2003; **425**:846-851

[53] Bailey JM, Swanson BJ, Hamada T, Eggers JP, Singh PK, Caffery T, et al. Sonic hedgehog promotes desmoplasia in pancreatic cancer. Clinical Cancer Research. 2008;**14**:5995-6004

[54] Feldmann G, Fendrich V, McGovern K, Bedja D, Bisht S, Alvarez H, et al. An orally bioavailable small-molecule inhibitor of hedgehog signaling inhibits tumor initiation and metastasis in pancreatic cancer. Molecular Cancer Therapeutics. 2008;**7**: 2725-2735

[55] Feldmann G, Habbe N, Dhara S, Bisht S, Alvarez H, Fendrich V, et al. Hedgehog inhibition prolongs survival in a genetically engineered mouse model of pancreatic cancer. Gut. 2008;**57**: 1420-1430

[56] Olive KP, Jacobetz MA, Davidson CJ, Gopinathan A, McIntyre D, Honess D, et al. Inhibition of hedgehog signaling enhances delivery of chemotherapy in a mouse model of pancreatic cancer. Science. 2009;**324**:1457-1461

[57] Rhim AD, Oberstein PE, Thomas DH, Mirek ET, Palermo CF, Sastra SA, et al. Stromal elements act to restrain, rather than support, pancreatic ductal adenocarcinoma. Cancer Cell. 2014;**25**(6):735-747

[58] Lee JJ, Perera RM, Wang H, Wu D-C, Liu XS, Han S, et al. Stromal response to hedgehog signaling restrains pancreatic cancer progression. Proceedings of the National Academy of Sciences of the United States of America. 2014;**111**:E3091-E3100

[59] Steele NG, Biffi G, Kemp SB, Zhang Y, Drouillard D, Syu L, et al. Inhibition of hedgehog signaling alters fibroblast composition in pancreatic cancer. Clinical Cancer Research. 2021; **27**(7):2023-2037. DOI: 10.1158/1078-0432.CCR-20-3715

[60] Kim EJ, Sahai V, Abel EV, Griffith KA, Greenson JK, Takebe N, et al. Pilot clinical trial of hedgehog pathway inhibitor GDC-0449 (vismodegib) in combination with gemcitabine in patients with metastatic pancreatic adenocarcinoma. Clinical Cancer Research. 2014;**20**(23): 5937-5945. DOI: 10.1158/1078-0432.CCR-14-1269

[61] Ko AH, LoConte N, Tempero MA, Walker EJ, Kate Kelley R, Lewis S, et al. A phase I study of FOLFIRINOX plus IPI-926, a hedgehog pathway inhibitor, for advanced pancreatic adenocarcinoma. Pancreas. 2016;**45**:370-375

[62] Quaglio D, Infante P, Di Marcotullio L, Botta B, Mori M. Hedgehog signaling pathway inhibitors: An updated patent review (2015-present). Expert Opinion on Therapeutic Patents. 2020;**30**(4):235-250. DOI: 10.1080/13543776.2020.1730327

[63] Incardona JP, Gaffield W, Kapur RP, Roelink H. The teratogenic Veratrum alkaloid cyclopamine inhibits sonic hedgehog signal transduction. Development. 1998;**125**:3553-3562

[64] Berman DM, Karhadkar SS, Hallahan AR, Pritchard JI, Eberhart CG, Watkins DN, et al. Medulloblastoma growth inhibition by hedgehog pathway blockade. Science. 2002;**297**:1559-1561

[65] Lin TL, Matsui W. Hedgehog pathway as a drug target: Smoothened inhibitors in development. Oncotargets and Therapy. 2012;**5**:47

[66] Sekulic A, Migden MR, Oro AE, Dirix L, Lewis KD, Hainsworth JD, et al. Efficacy and safety of Vismodegib in advanced basal-cell carcinoma. The New England Journal of Medicine. 2012;**366**: 2171-2179

[67] Sekulic A, Migden MR, Basset-Seguin N, Garbe C, Gesierich A, Lao CD, et al. Long-term safety and efficacy of vismodegib in patients with advanced basal cell carcinoma: Final update of the pivotal ERIVANCE BCC study. BMC Cancer. 2017;**17**:332

[68] Pan S, Wu X, Jiang J, Gao W, Wan Y, Cheng D, et al. Discovery of NVP-LDE225, a potent and selective smoothened antagonist. ACS Medicinal Chemistry Letters. 2010;**1**(3):130-134. DOI: 10.1021/ml1000307

[69] Migden MR, Guminski A, Gutzmer R, Dirix L, Lewis KD, Combemale P, et al. Treatment with two different doses of sonidegib in patients with locally advanced or metastatic basal cell carcinoma (BOLT): A multicentre, randomised, double-blind phase 2 trial. The Lancet Oncology. 2015; **16**(6):716-728. DOI: 10.1016/S1470-2045(15)70100-2

[70] Munchhof MJ, Li Q, Shavnya A, Borzillo GV, Boyden TL, Jones CS, et al. Discovery of PF-04449913, a potent and orally bioavailable inhibitor of smoothened. ACS Medicinal Chemistry Letters. 2012;**3**:106-111

[71] Cortes JE, Heidel FH, Hellmann A, Fiedler W, Smith BD, Robak T, et al.

Randomized comparison of low dose cytarabine with or without glasdegib in patients with newly diagnosed acute myeloid leukemia or high-risk myelodysplastic syndrome. Leukemia. 2019;**33**:379-389

[72] Chang ALS, Oro AE. Initial assessment of tumor regrowth after Vismodegib in advanced basal cell carcinoma. Archives of Dermatology. 2012;**148**:1324-1325

[73] Jain R, Dubey SK, Singhvi G. The hedgehog pathway and its inhibitors: Emerging therapeutic approaches for basal cell carcinoma. Drug Discovery Today. 2022;**27**(4):1176-1183. DOI: 10.1016/j.drudis.2021.12.005

[74] Yao CD, Haensel D, Gaddam S, Patel T, Atwood SX, Sarin KY, et al. AP-1 and TGFß cooperativity drives non-canonical hedgehog signaling in resistant basal cell carcinoma. Nature Communications. 2020;**11**:5079

[75] Whitson RJ, Lee A, Urman NM, Mirza A, Yao CY, Brown AS, et al. Noncanonical hedgehog pathway activation through SRF–MKL1 promotes drug resistance in basal cell carcinomas. Nature Medicine. 2018;**24**:271-281

[76] Zhao X, Ponomaryov T, Ornell KJ, Zhou P, Dabral SK, Pak E, et al. RAS/MAPK activation drives resistance to Smo inhibition, metastasis, and tumor evolution in Shh pathway–dependent tumors. Cancer Research. 2015;**75**:3623-3635

[77] Sharpe HJ, Pau G, Dijkgraaf GJ, Gerrit J, Basset-Seguin N, Modrusan Z, et al. Genomic analysis of smoothened inhibitor resistance in basal cell carcinoma. Cancer Cell. 2015;**27**:327-341

[78] Zhao X, Pak E, Ornell KJ, Pazyra-Murphy MF, Mac Kenzie EL, Chadwick EJ, et al. Transposon screen identifies loss of primary cilia as a mechanism of resistance to SMO inhibitors. Cancer Discovery. 2017;**7**:1436-1449

[79] Infante P, Mori M, Alfonsi R, et al. Gli1/DNA interaction is a druggable target for hedgehog-dependent tumors. The EMBO Journal. 2015;**34**:200-217

[80] Atwood SX, Sarin KY, Whitson RJ, Li JR, Kim G, Rezaee M, et al. Smoothened variants explain the majority of drug resistance in basal cell carcinoma. Cancer Cell. 2015;**27**:342-353. DOI: 10.1016/j.ccell.2015.02.002

[81] Zhang M, Gao L, Ye Y, Li X. Advances in glioma-associated oncogene (GLI) inhibitors for cancer therapy. Investigational New Drugs. 2022;**40**(2):370-388. DOI: 10.1007/s10637-021-01187-2

[82] The Nobel Prize in Physiology or Medicine. 2018. Available from: https://www.nobelprize.org/prizes/medicine/2018/summary/

[83] Dammeijer F, van Gulijk M, Mulder EE, Lukkes M, Klaase L, van den Bosch T, et al. The PD-1/PD-L1-checkpoint restrains T cell immunity in tumor-draining lymph nodes. Cancer Cell. 2020;**38**(5):685-700.e8. DOI: 10.1016/j.ccell.2020.09.001

[84] Chang ALS, Tran DC, Cannon JGD, Li S, Jeng M, Patel R, et al. Pembrolizumab for advanced basal cell carcinoma: An investigator-initiated, proof- of-concept study. Journal of the American Academy of Dermatology. 2019;**80**(2):564-566. DOI: 10.1016/j.jaad.2018.08.017

[85] Dummer R, Guminksi A, Gutzmer R, Lear JT, Lewis KD, Chang ALS, et al. Long-term efficacy

and safety of sonidegib in patients with advanced basal cell carcinoma: 42-month analysis of the phase II randomized, double-blind BOLT study. The British Journal of Dermatology. 2020;**182**(6): 1369-1378. DOI: 10.1111/bjd.18552

[86] FDA approves cemiplimab-rwlc for locally advanced and metastatic basal cell carcinoma. Available from: https://www.fda.gov/drugs/resources-information-approved-drugs/fda-approves-cemiplimab-rwlc-locally-advanced-and-metastatic-basal-cell-carcinoma

[87] Stratigos AJ, Sekulic A, Peris K, et al. Cemiplimab in locally advanced basal cell carcinoma after hedgehog inhibitor therapy: An open-label, multi-Centre, single-arm, phase 2 trial. The Lancet Oncology. 2021;**22**:848-857

[88] Gambichler T, Stricker I, Neid M, Tannapfel A, Susok L. Impressive response to four cemiplimab cycles of a sonidegib-resistant giant basosquamous carcinoma of the midface. Journal of the European Academy of Dermatology and Venereology. 2022;**36**(6):e490-e492. DOI: 10.1111/jdv.17993

[89] Grund-Gröschke S, Stockmaier G, Aberger F. Hedgehog/GLI signaling in tumor immunity - new therapeutic opportunities and clinical implications. Cell Communication and Signaling: CCS. 2019;**17**(1):172. DOI: 10.1186/s12964-019-0459-7

[90] de la Roche M, Ritter AT, Angus KL, Dinsmore C, Earnshaw CH, Reiter JF, et al. Hedgehog signaling controls T cell killing at the immunological synapse. Science. 2013;**342**(6163):1247-1250. DOI: 10.1126/science.1244689

Chapter 7

Perspective Chapter: Role of Cancer-Associated Fibroblasts in Oncogenesis

Anyu Gu, Chikezie O. Madu and Yi Lu

Abstract

The tumor microenvironment consists of multiple types of cells, including endothelial cells, pericytes, neutrophil macrophage mast cells, lymphatic cells, basement membrane extracellular matrix, as well as fibroblasts. Fibroblasts populations found in cancers, also known as cancer-associated fibroblasts, have been implicated in the initiation, progression, and metastasis of tumors. This chapter will focus on the roles of cancer-associated fibroblasts in the progression of cancer and the studies of use of cancer-associated fibroblasts as a therapeutic target for cancer intervention.

Keywords: tumor microenvironment, cancer-associated fibroblasts, fibroblasts, cancer intervention, cancer

1. Introduction

The tumor microenvironment (TME) is the environment in which tumor cells or cancer stem cells exist [1]. The TME consists of multiple types of cells, including endothelial cells, immune cells, and fibroblasts [1–3]. The TME also consists of components such as the extracellular matrix (ECM), soluble factors such as cytokines and growth factors, and physical properties such as pH and oxygen content [2]. The TME and the interactions between its components help to promote tumor growth and cancer progression (**Figure 1**) [3].

Fibroblasts are the most common type of cell in connective tissue, commonly defined as structural cells that specialize in depositing and remodeling the ECM [4]. Fibroblast populations found in primary and metastatic cancers, known as cancer-associated fibroblasts (CAFs), are implicated in tumor initiation, progression, and metastasis [5]. CAFs have wide varieties of cells-of-origin, heterogeneous phenotypes, and diverse functions, all of which are shared by other cells found in the TME [6]. This chapter will focus on CAFs and their potential use in cancer intervention.

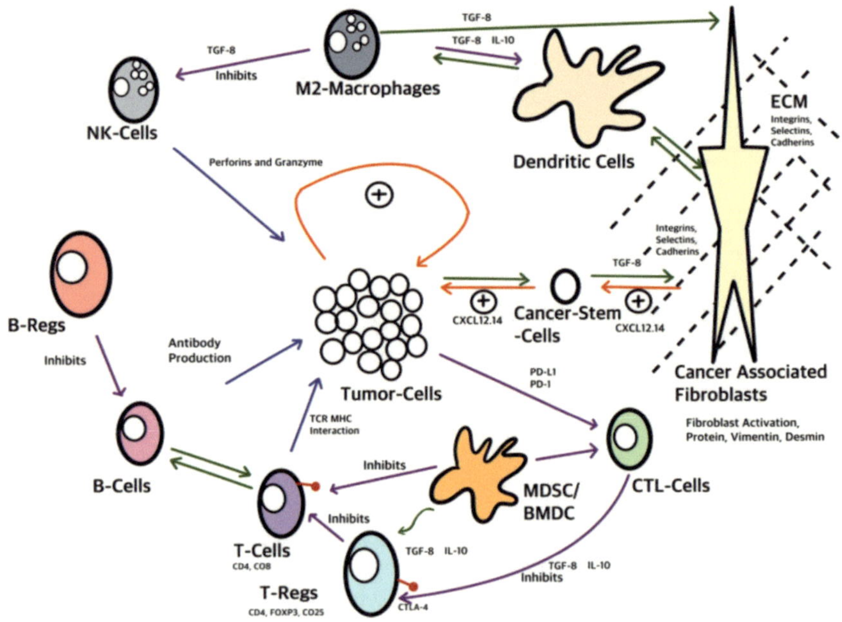

Figure 1.
Important interactions and mechanisms of the TME [1].

2. Fibroblasts and cancer-associated fibroblasts

The precursors of CAFs are generally considered to be dormant tissue-resident fibroblasts and pancreatic and hepatic stellate cells, though different studies have also identified bone marrow-derived mesenchymal stem cells, endothelial cells, and adipocytes [5]. Fibroblasts play a prominent role in coordinating the wound repair response in skin; therefore, it is likely that key CAF traits correspond to the normal physiological role normal fibroblasts play [7]. Fibroblasts transform into CAFs through tumor-derived stimuli, including soluble factors secreted by the tumor, immune infiltrate, lysophosphatidic acid, fibroblast growth factor, interleukin-1 (IL-1), IL-6, and granulin [8]. Transforming growth factor β (TGFβ) and lysophosphatidic acid are well-established activating signals for fibroblasts, which promote the activity of SMAD transcription factors and serum response factors, respectively [7]. These fibroblast activating signals converge to drive expression of the fibroblast marker αSMA, as well as increase the activity of the contractile cytoskeleton [7]. Fibroblasts may become activated through Notch signaling when in direct contact with tumor cells [7, 8]. Other mechanisms that can activate normal fibroblasts to become CAFs are shown in **Figure 2**. In the TME, tumor cells secrete factors such as TGFβ, platelet-derived growth factor (PGDF), and fibroblast growth factor (FGF) to convert fibroblasts to CAFs [3]. A build-up of CAFs is often associated with poor prognosis in many cancer types [3].

As shown in **Figure 3** [10], TGFβ is a common factor in the conversion of many different cell types into fibroblasts and CAFs. There are many types of TGFβ. TGFβ-1 is one that is secreted by stromal and tumor cells and is the main factor in promoting the mobilization of residential fibroblasts and their activation into CAFs [10]. Through SMAD-dependent and SMAD-independent pathways, TGFβ-1 activates fibroblasts into CAFs, expressing alpha-smooth muscle actin, periostin, α-fibroblast

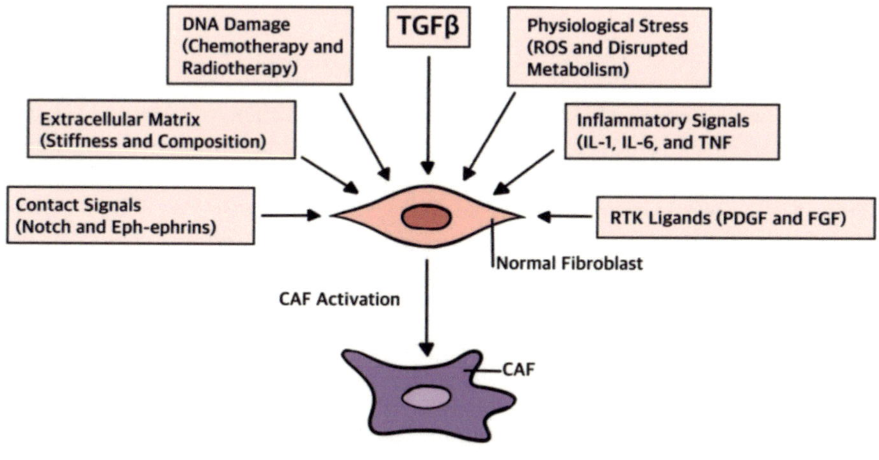

Figure 2.
Mechanisms that activate normal fibroblasts to become CAFs. FGF, fibroblast growth factor; PDGF, platelet-derived growth factor; ROS, reactive oxygen species; RTK, receptor tyrosine kinase; TGFβ, transforming growth factor-β; TNF, tumor necrosis factor [7].

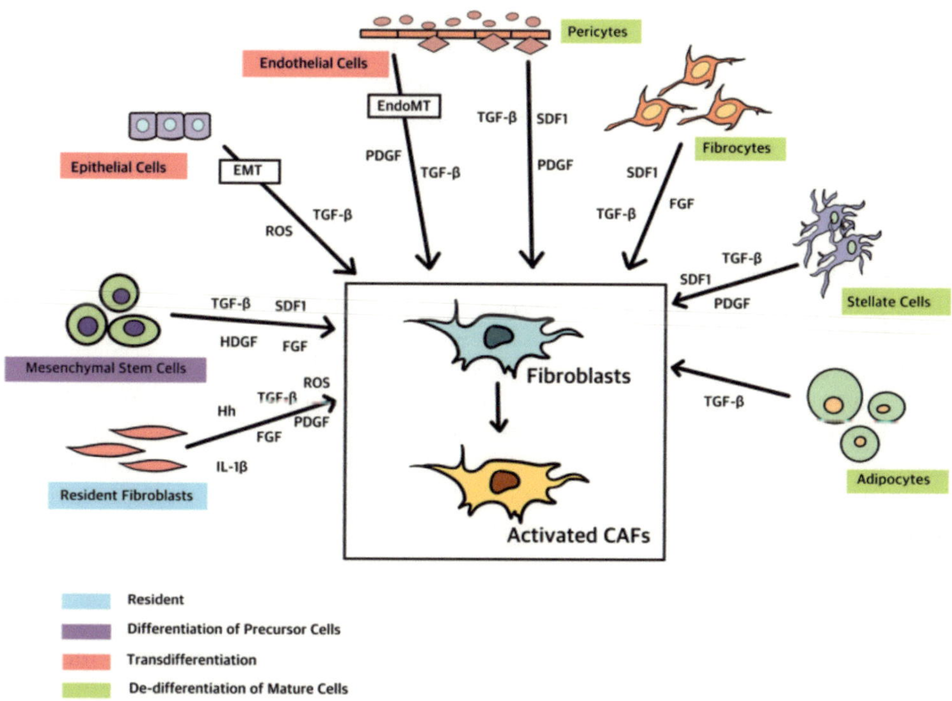

Figure 3.
Different origins of CAFs [9, 10].

activation protein, and fibroblast-specific protein-1 [10]. In addition, activated fibroblasts secrete TGFβ-1 [10], which could create a positive feedback loop, increasing fibroblast activation. TGFβ binds to the type 2 of TGFβ receptor (TGFBR2) on the surface of fibroblasts [11].

2.1 CAFs in tumors

CAFs are a type of myofibroblast that enhance the malignancy and progression of cancer [12]. The presence of CAFs is identified in almost all solid tumors [13]. This suggests that CAFs are important to the formation of solid tumors. In an established tumor, the TME represents a changed part of the original normal tissue of the host [13]. Tumor cells mostly contribute to the change in their favor. [13]. The stromal transformation of TME is primarily dominated and maintained by CAFs [13]. The CAF component of the TME is the most critical in influencing most of the functions of the TME in real time [13]. CAFs alter the TME by directly interacting with cancer cells and regulatory paracrine signaling, control the immune response to neoplasia, deposit ECM components, stimulate angiogenesis, and provide a scaffold for tumor invasion and metastasis [14]. Additionally, CAFs can produce many growth factors and pro-inflammatory cytokines to promote angiogenesis and recruit immunosuppressive cells to the TME to evade the immune system [9].

While CAFs have historically been considered to be cancer-promoting components, recent studies have shown that CAFs could have tumor-restraining functions in certain circumstances [15]. The tumor-restraining actions of CAFs are likely dependent on stimulation of anticancer immunity, pro-inflammatory secretome, tumor inhibitory signaling, and the synthesis of ECM components as barriers to tumor cell invasion and dissemination [5]. A study in mice has shown that myofibroblast depletion leads to increased tumor invasion, which is associated with decreased survival [16]. This study suggests that CAFs have functions in restraining tumors. This paradoxical nature of CAFs can potentially be explained by the heterogeneity of CAFs [15].

2.2 Heterogeneity of CAFs

There is mounting evidence that CAFs are a heterogeneous population of cells [9]. This likely depends on the numerous precursors of CAFs [9]. CAFs can be recruited to the tumor from a distant source, such as bone marrow [14], or transdifferentiate from non-fibroblastic lineages, such as epithelial cells, blood vessels, adipocytes, pericytes, and smooth muscle cells [9]. Numerous precursors of CAFs are shown in **Figure 3**. The study of genetically modified mouse models (GEMMs) designed to limit the accumulation of CAFs in growing pancreatic tumors or to conditionally delete the vascular endothelial growth factors in breast CAFs revealed that there are distinct functional subtypes of CAFs [17].

2.3 Functions of CAFs

CAFs have both pro-tumor and antitumor tendencies [17]. Pro-tumorigenic functions of CAFs are generally driven by their altered secretive [17]. Paracrine signaling between cancer cells and CAFs leads to tumor progression by enhancing the survival, proliferation, stemness, and metastasis-initiating capacity of cancer cells, promoting cancer progression and enhancing resistance to therapy [17]. CAFs also have an indirect influence in promoting tumor growth due to their ability to remodel the ECM [17]. The stiffness of the tissue, which plays a critical role in tumorigenesis, is influenced by modifications in the ECM's composition and cross-linking [18, 19]. CAFs express lysyl oxidase (LOX), an enzyme that cross-links and stiffens collagen fibers, promoting their stability [18]. CAFs also regulate the degradation of the ECM

[18]. CAFs secrete cytokines and chemokines that regulate tumor immunity and the intratumoral vascular program [17]. Several studies have indicated that CAFs play an important role in chemoresistance *via* different mechanisms, including but not limited to increasing stem cancer cells, secreting cytokines, and secreting miRNAs [10]. miRNAs have been shown to inhibit tumor-repressor genes, thus promoting cell growth and invasion, metastasis, and tumorigenesis [20].

CAFs trigger tumor initiation and progression [18]. *In vitro* coculture and *in vivo* transplantation experiments have shown that human prostatic CAFs induced the proliferation and the ability to form tumors from immortalized nontumorigenic human prostatic epithelial cells [18]. This effect was not exhibited by normal fibroblasts. It is thought that CAFs' secreted factors are what cause this tumor-initiating potential [18].

Numerous studies have shown that CAFs confer resistance to chemotherapy [6]. Some CAF-mediated resistant mechanisms include delivery of exosomes stimulating cancer cell survival, promoting cancer cell epithelial-mesenchymal transition, and thus decreasing expression of transporters responsible for drug uptake and scavenging chemo drug to reduce the amount of intratumoral chemotherapy drug [6]. CAFs also contribute to the resistance to targeted therapy [6]. Additionally, evidence suggests that CAFs contribute to immune evasion and immunotherapy resistance [6].

Antitumor functions of CAFs are predominantly associated with their functions as regulators of antitumor immunity [17]. Studies in mice have shown that fibroblast depletion leads to increased tumor invasion [16]. The use of defined gene promoter-driven expression of viral thymidine kinase proteins in GEMMs to study CAFs has allowed researchers to deplete populations of CAFs using ganciclovir, a substance that is toxic only to cells that express viral thymidine kinase [17]. A similar approach to deplete CAFs expressing αSMA suggested that αSMA+ stromal cells were predominantly acting to restrain cancer progression [17]. The depletion of these αSMA expressing CAFs yielded a more invasive tumor with enhanced intratumoral hypoxia [17]. A reduction in CAFs in GEMMs of pancreatic tumors with a deletion of sonic hedgehog (SHH) in the cancer cells also resulted in more aggressive tumors with increased cancer proliferation [17].

3. Targeting CAFs for cancer intervention

Numerous studies have proven CAFs' significant role in cancer progression and subsequently the potential of CAFs as targets for effective cancer intervention. Traditionally, therapies involved targeting cancer cells directly [21]. Recent complementary efforts aim to disrupt the networks that promote cancer cell activity and behavior [21]. The depletion of CAFs and targeting of CAF-dependent pathways can indirectly result in malignant cell death through both immune-dependent and immune-independent mechanisms [21]. Most conventional cancer therapies, such as radiotherapy and chemotherapy, are likely to affect CAFs as well by preventing cellular division by inducing DNA damage, impeding DNA and RNA synthesis, and blocking the cytoskeleton remodel required for cell division [17]. However, the unintended impact of these therapeutic methods on the function and accumulation of CAFs is largely unknown [17].

As a result, research is being conducted to help target CAFs through alternative methods [21]. One approach involves targeting the regulatory pathways leading to fibroblast differentiation and activation [9, 17, 21]. For example, TGFβ is a common

Drugs	Target and mechanism	Cancer types	National Clinical Trial number	Status	Ref.
Sibrotuzumab	131I-labeled anti-FAP mAb	Colorectal, non-small cell lung, breast, or head and neck cancers	NCT02198274 NCT02209727	Phase I	[24]
Calcipotriol Paricalcitol	Vitamin D analogue	Early-stage skin cancer, breast cancer, pancreatic cancer	NCT03596073 NCT04617067 NCT02030860 NCT03138720 NCT04054362	Phase I/II	[25]
Pamrevlumab (FG-3019)	Anti-CTGF mAb	Pancreatic cancer	NCT03941093	Phase III	[26]
Plerixafor (AMD3100) BL-8040 (motixafortide)	CXCR4 receptor antagonist	Pancreatic cancer	NCT04177810 NCT02179970 NCT02826486 NCT03193190	Phase I/II	[27, 28]
IPI-926	Smoothened inhibitor	Pancreatic cancer	NCT01130142	Phase I	[29]
S-3304	MMP inhibitor	Advanced solid tumors	NCT00078390 NCT00033215	Phase I	[30]
131I-m81C6	131I-labeled anti-tenascin mAb	Brain tumors	NCT00002752 NCT00003461	Phase II	[31]
Imatinib	PDGFR inhibitor	Advanced solid tumors	NCT00161213 NCT00281996 NCT01048320 NCT00485485	Phase I/II	[32]
GS-6624 (simtuzumab)	LOXL2 mAb	Pancreatic cancer	NCT01472198 NCT01479465	Phase II	[33]
Tetrathiomolybdate	Copper chelator, target LOX	Breast cancer, prostate cancer	NCT00195091 NCT00150995 NCT00405574	Phase II	[34]
Pegvorhyaluronidase alfa (PEGPH20; PVHA)	Recombinant human hyaluronidase	Lung cancer, pancreatic cancer	NCT01453153 NCT02563548 NCT01839487 NCT02715804	Phase I/ II/III	

Table 1.
Summary of various drugs' efficacy against CAF-induced cancer progression in clinical and pre-clinical studies [6].

factor in the conversion of different cell types into CAFs. In a study, Mariathasan et al. found the two top scoring TGFβ pathway genes represent a ligand, TGFβ1, and receptor TGFβR2 [22]. In murine tumor models, blocking the TGFβ signaling by using the SM16 TGFβ receptor inhibitor or anti-TGFβ antibodies resulted in the recession of tumor growth [23]. By targeting these regulatory pathways, the activation of fibroblasts could be prevented, preventing CAFs from activating and functioning.

Another approach for targeting CAFs for cancer intervention is targeting CAF-secreted factors [11]. Numerous mitogens, chemokines, and matricellular proteins that CAFs release aid in the evolution of tumor progression and the development of drug resistance [11]. Targeting these CAF-secreted factors should prevent the promotion of tumor progression and drug resistance, making the tumor more susceptible to drugs. The heterogeneity of CAFs also proves as an advantage for cancer intervention *via* shifting the influence of pro- vs. antitumorigenic populations [21].

Currently, there are many drugs under trial as shown in **Table 1**. Of the potential targets identified in CAFs, fibroblast-activation protein (FAP) is the most studied. FAP has been neither detected in benign tumors nor in most normal quiescent adult stromal cells [35]. FAP is a type II integral membrane of the prolyl oligopeptidase family, or S9 family [36]. FAP is further classified into the dipeptidyl peptidase (DPP) subfamily (S9B) [36]. This class of enzymes is characterized by its capacity to cleave the pro-Xaa peptide link, where Xaa can be any amino acid. It has been demonstrated that this enzymatic activity contributes to the development of cancer by altering bioactive signaling peptides [36]. *In vivo,* FAP+ CAFs were successfully depleted by the FAP-depleting immunotoxin, and tumor models demonstrated strong tumor inhibitory effects. [6]. Other approaches in targeting FAP include DNA vaccine and chimeric antigen receptor (CAR) T cells [6].

4. Conclusions

Heterogeneous populations of CAFs exist in the TME. The heterogeneous nature of CAFs likely comes from their different origins, and this heterogeneity is likely the cause of the paradoxical nature of CAFs having both pro-tumorigenic and antitumorigenic functions. CAFs have many functions in the TME. CAFs alter the TME. They produce growth factors and pro-inflammatory cytokines.

CAFs are a promising target for cancer intervention. They have many pro-tumorigenic functions. CAFs can be targeted through their activation pathway by blocking a step in the pathway. One method is by preventing FAP from being produced by introducing siRNAs that are complementary to the FAP mRNA.

Over time, our understanding of CAFs and their contribution to cancer progression has expanded greatly. We now have a better understanding of their heterogeneity and their functions in the TME. While the antitumorigenic functions may act as a roadblock to targeting CAFs for cancer intervention, it may be possible to develop a treatment that targets the pro-tumorigenic functions of CAFs without targeting the antitumorigenic functions of CAFs by targeting subpopulations of CAFs that express pro-tumorigenic genes.

While CAFs are a promising target for cancer intervention due to their pro-tumorigenic functions, their antitumorigenic functions may act as a roadblock. Further research would be required before targeting CAFs as a conventional method of cancer intervention.

However, there are issues with targeting CAFs for cancer intervention. **Figure 4** shows the effects of targeting only tumor cells vs. targeting only the TME on a tumor. In both, there is a possibility that the tumor can grow back. In addition, studies in mice have shown that fibroblast depletion leads to increased tumor invasion [16]. In mouse models, deletion of SHH accelerated the progression of pancreatic ductal adenocarcinoma [37].

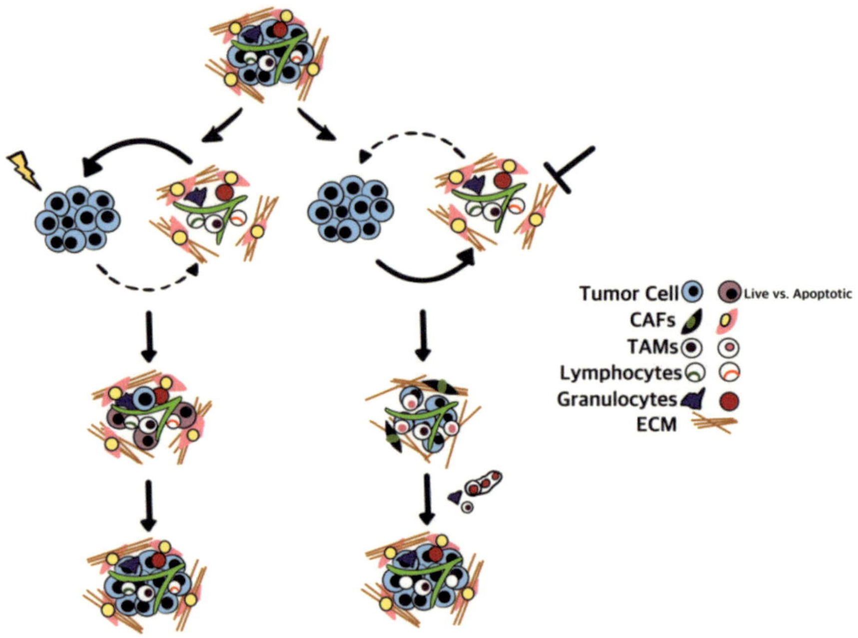

Figure 4.
A schematic diagram of targeting tumor cell or TME only and their potential resistance mechanisms. Left: Targeting tumor cells only (such as chemotherapies) kills majority tumor cells. However, the residue tumor cells may survive due to the TME, leading to tumor relapse. Right: Targeting the TME can inhibit the recruitment and activation of pro-tumor cells and enhance antitumor responses. However, the TME will be reconstituted by tumor cells via recruitment and programming of bone marrow derived cells or local resident stromal or immune cells [6].

Acknowledgements

Funding for the publication of this paper was made possible by a grant from The Assisi Foundation of Memphis. Brown, Chester, PhD (PI). We also thank Yirui Tang for drawing the figures used in this paper.

Conflict of interest

The authors have declared that no conflict of interest exists.

Author details

Anyu Gu[1], Chikezie O. Madu[2] and Yi Lu[3*]

1 Departments of Biology, White Station High, Memphis, TN, USA

2 Departments of Biological Sciences, University of Memphis, Memphis, TN, USA

3 Department of Pathology and Laboratory Medicine, University of Tennessee Health Science Center, Memphis, Tennessee, USA

*Address all correspondence to: ylu@utshc.edu

References

[1] Arneth B. Tumor microenvironment. Medicina. 2019;**56**(1):15

[2] Soysal SD, Tzankov A, Muenst SE. Role of the tumor microenvironment in breast cancer. Pathobiology. 2015;**82**(3-4):142-152

[3] Anderson NM, Simon MC. The tumor microenvironment. Current Biology. 2020;**30**(16):R921-R925. DOI: 10.1016/j.cub.2020.06.081 PMID: 32810447; PMCID: PMC8194051

[4] Kirk T, Ahmed A, Rognoni E. Fibroblast memory in development, homeostasis and disease. Cell. 2021;**10**(11):2840

[5] Chen Y, McAndrews KM, Kalluri R. Clinical and therapeutic relevance of cancer-associated fibroblasts. Nature Reviews Clinical Oncology. 2021;**18**(12):792-804

[6] Xiao Y, Yu D. Tumor microenvironment as a therapeutic target in cancer. Pharmacology & Therapeutics. 2021;**221**:107753

[7] Sahai E, Astsaturov I, Cukierman E, DeNardo DG, Egeblad M, Evans RM, et al. A framework for advancing our understanding of cancer-associated fibroblasts. Nature Reviews Cancer. 2020;**20**(3):174-186

[8] Park D, Sahai E, Rullan A. SnapShot: Cancer-associated fibroblasts. Cell. 2020;**181**(2):486-486.e1. DOI: 10.1016/j.cell.2020.03.013 PMID: 32302576

[9] Liu T, Han C, Wang S, Fang P, Ma Z, Xu L, et al. Cancer-associated fibroblasts: An emerging target of anti-cancer immunotherapy. Journal of Hematology & Oncology. 2019;**12**(1):1-15

[10] Louault K, Li RR, DeClerck YA. Cancer-associated fibroblasts: Understanding their heterogeneity. Cancers. 2020;**12**(11):3108

[11] Öhlund D, Elyada E, Tuveson D. Fibroblast heterogeneity in the cancer wound. Journal of Experimental Medicine. 2014;**211**(8):1503-1523

[12] Tang PC, Chung JY, Xue VW, Xiao J, Meng XM, Huang XR, et al. Smad3 promotes Cancer-associated fibroblasts generation via macrophage-Myofibroblast transition. Advanced Science. 2022;**9**(1):e2101235. DOI: 10.1002/advs.202101235 PMID: 34791825; PMCID: PMC8728853

[13] De P, Aske J, Dey N. Cancer-associated fibroblast functions as a road-block in Cancer therapy. Cancers. 2021;**13**(20):5246

[14] Yoshida GJ. Regulation of heterogeneous cancer-associated fibroblasts: The molecular pathology of activated signaling pathways. Journal of Experimental & Clinical Cancer Research. 2020;**39**(1):1-15

[15] Biffi G, Tuveson DA. Diversity and biology of cancer-associated fibroblasts. Physiological Reviews. 2021;**101**(1):147-176

[16] Özdemir BC, Pentcheva-Hoang T, Carstens JL, Zheng X, Wu CC, Simpson TR, et al. Depletion of carcinoma-associated fibroblasts and fibrosis induces immunosuppression and accelerates pancreas cancer with reduced survival. Cancer Cell. 2014;**25**(6):719-734

[17] LeBleu VS, Kalluri R. A peek into cancer-associated fibroblasts: Origins, functions and translational impact.

Disease Models & Mechanisms. 2018;**11**(4):dmm029447

[18] Pickup MW, Laklai H, Acerbi I, Owens P, Gorska AE, Chytil A, et al. Stromally derived Lysyl oxidase promotes metastasis of transforming growth factor-β–deficient mouse mammary CarcinomasStromal LOX promotes TGFβR2-null breast Cancer metastasis. Cancer Research. 2013;**73**(17):5336-5346

[19] Cukierman, E., & Bassi, D. E. (2010). Physico-mechanical aspects of extracellular matrix influences on tumorigenic behaviors. In Seminars in cancer Biology (Vol. 20, No. 3, pp. 139-145). Academic Press.

[20] Madu CO, Gu A, Madu C, Lu Y. The Role of MicroRNAs in the Progression, Prognostication, and Treatment of Breast Cancer. 2020

[21] Barrett RL, Puré E. Cancer-associated fibroblasts and their influence on tumor immunity and immunotherapy. eLife. 2020;**9**:e57243

[22] Mariathasan S et al. TGFβ attenuates tumour response to PD-L1 blockade by contributing to exclusion of T cells. Nature. 2018;**554**(7693):544-548. DOI: 10.1038/nature25501. Epub 2018 Feb 14

[23] Zhao H et al. Inflammation and tumor progression: Signaling pathways and targeted intervention. Signal Transduction and Targeted Therapy. 2021;**6**(1):263. DOI: 10.1038/s41392-021-00658-5

[24] Siveke JT. Fibroblast-activating protein: Targeting the roots of the tumor microenvironment. Journal of Nuclear Medicine. 2018;**59**:1412-1414. DOI: 10.2967/jnumed.118.214361

[25] Sherman MH et al. Vitamin D receptor-mediated stromal reprogramming suppresses pancreatitis and enhances pancreatic cancer therapy. Cell. 2014;**159**:80-93. DOI: 10.1016/j.cell.2014.08.007

[26] Neesse A et al. CTGF antagonism with mAb FG-3019 enhances chemotherapy response without increasing drug delivery in murine ductal pancreas cancer. Proceedings of the National Academy of Sciences of the United States of America. 2013;**110**:12325-12330. DOI: 10.1073/pnas.1300415110

[27] Feig C et al. Targeting CXCL12 from FAP-expressing carcinoma-associated fibroblasts synergizes with anti-PD-L1 immunotherapy in pancreatic cancer. Proceedings of the National Academy of Sciences of the United States of America. 2013;**110**:20212-20217. DOI: 10.1073/pnas.1320318110

[28] Bockorny B et al. BL-8040, a CXCR4 antagonist, in combination with pembrolizumab and chemotherapy for pancreatic cancer: The COMBAT trial. Nature Medicine. 2020;**26**:878-+. DOI: 10.1038/s41591-020-0880-x

[29] Jimeno A et al. Phase I study of the hedgehog pathway inhibitor IPI-926 in adult patients with solid tumors. Clinical Cancer Research. 2013;**19**:2766-2774. DOI: 10.1158/1078-0432.CCR-12-3654

[30] Chiappori AA et al. A phase I pharmacokinetic and pharmacodynamic study of s-3304, a novel matrix metalloproteinase inhibitor, in patients with advanced and refractory solid tumors. Clinical Cancer Research. 2007;**13**:2091-2099. DOI: 10.1158/1078-0432.CCR-06-1586

[31] Reardon DA et al. Salvage radioimmunotherapy with murine iodine-131-labeled antitenascin monoclonal antibody 81C6 for patients

with recurrent primary and metastatic malignant brain tumors: Phase II study results. Journal of Clinical Oncology. 2006;**24**:115-122. DOI: 10.1200/JCO.2005.03.4082

[32] Reilley MJ et al. Phase I clinical trial of combination imatinib and ipilimumab in patients with advanced malignancies. Journal for Immunotherapy of Cancer. 2017;**5**:35. DOI: 10.1186/s40425-017-0238-1

[33] Benson AB 3rd et al. A phase II randomized, double-blind, placebo-controlled study of Simtuzumab or placebo in combination with gemcitabine for the first-line treatment of pancreatic adenocarcinoma. The Oncologist. 2017;**22**:e241-e215. DOI: 10.1634/theoncologist.2017-0024

[34] Chan N et al. Influencing the tumor microenvironment: A phase II study of copper depletion using Tetrathiomolybdate in patients with breast Cancer at high risk for recurrence and in preclinical models of lung metastases. Clinical Cancer Research. 2017;**23**:666-676. DOI: 10.1158/1078-0432.CCR-16-13261078-0432.CCR-16-1326 [pii]

[35] Wang LCS, Lo A, Scholler J, Sun J, Majumdar RS, Kapoor V, et al. Targeting fibroblast activation protein in tumor stroma with chimeric antigen receptor T cells can inhibit tumor growth and augment host immunity without severe ToxicityFAP-redirected CAR T cells. Cancer Immunology Research. 2014;**2**(2):154-166

[36] Brennen WN, Isaacs JT, Denmeade SR. Rationale behind targeting fibroblast activation protein–expressing carcinoma-associated fibroblasts as a novel chemotherapeutic strategy. Molecular Cancer Therapeutics. 2012;**11**(2):257-266

[37] Rhim AD, Oberstein PE, Thomas DH, Mirek ET, Palermo CF, Sastra SA, et al. Stromal elements act to restrain, rather than support, pancreatic ductal adenocarcinoma. Cancer Cell. 2014;**25**(6):735-747